VAGUS NERVE

Improve the quality of your life. Discover the Vagus nerve's functions and self-help exercises to reduce anxiety, depression, PTSD, and lots more.

The information herein is offered for informational purposes solely, and is universal as so. The presentation of the information is without contract or any type of guarantee assurance.

The trademarks that are used are without any consent, and the publication of the trademark is without permission or backing by the trademark owner. All trademarks and brands within this book are for clarifying purposes only and are the owned by the owners themselves, not affiliated with this document.

DISCLAIMER

All erudition contained in this book is given for informational and educational purposes only. The author is not, in any way, accountable for any results or outcomes that emanate from using this material. Constructive attempts have been made to provide information that is both accurate and effective, but the author is not bound for the accuracy or use/misuse of this information.

FOREWORD

First, I will like to thank you for taking the first step of trusting me and deciding to purchase/read this life-transforming eBook. Thanks for spending your time and resources on this material.

I can assure you of exact results if you will diligently follow the exact blueprint- I lay bare in the information manual you are currently reading. It has transformed lives, and I strongly believe it will equally transform your own life too.

All the information I presented in this Do-It-Yourself piece is easy to digest and practice.

TABLE OF CONTENTS

CHAPTER ONE

THE VAGUE NERVE: LOCATION, FUNCTIONS, AND IMPORTANCE

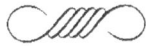

In cranial nerve, the vagus nerve seems to be the longest. It contains engine and tangible filaments and, in light of the fact that it goes through the neck and thorax to the belly, has the most extensive appropriation in the body. It contains substantial and instinctive afferent strands, just as general and uncommon instinctive efferent filaments.

It also happens to be the tenth cranial nerve - (CN X). It is a practically assorted nerve, offering a wide range of modalities of innervation. It is related with the subsidiaries of the fourth and sixth pharyngeal curves. Be aware that there are 12 cranial nerves in the body. They come in pairs and help to interface the cerebrum with various areas of the body, for instance, the head, neck, and center.

There are different sensory system capacities given

by the vagus nerve and its related parts. The vagus nerve capacities add to the autonomic sensory system, which comprises of the parasympathetic and thoughtful parts. The nerve is liable for certain tactile exercises and engine data for development inside the body.

Basically, it is a piece of a circuit that connects the neck, heart, lungs, and the guts to the mind. Some send actual data, including insights concerning smells, sights, tastes, and sounds, to the mind. These nerves are known as having material limits. Other cranial nerves control the improvement of various muscles and the limit of explicit organs. These are known as motor limits.

While some cranial nerves have either tactile or engine capacities, others have both. The vagus nerve is an example. The cranial nerves are characterized utilizing Roman numerals dependent on their area. The vagus nerve is additionally called cranial nerve X.

"Vagus" signifies "meandering" in Latin. This is an exceptionally proper name, as the vagus nerve is the longest cranial nerve. It runs right from the cerebrum stem to part of the colon.

The tactile elements of the vagus nerve are isolated into two segments:

- Somatic parts. Sensations that happen in the muscles or on the skin.

- Visceral parts. Sensations that happen in the other parts of the body.

- Tactile elements of the vagus nerve include:

- providing physical sensation data for the skin behind the ear, the outer piece of the ear channel, and certain parts of the throat.

- supplying instinctive sensation data for the larynx, throat, lungs, trachea, heart, and the majority of the stomach-related tract.

- playing a little activity in the vibe of taste near the establishment of the tongue.

- Motor components of the vagus nerve include:

- stimulating muscles in the pharynx, larynx, and the fragile feeling of taste, which is the bulky zone close to the back of the highest point of the mouth.

- stimulating muscles in the heart, where it cuts down resting beat.

- stimulating programmed compressions in the stomach-related tract, including the throat, stomach, and most by far of the stomach-related organs, which empower sustenance to go through the tract

Review:

- Sensory: Innervates the skin of the outer acoustic meatus and the inside surfaces of the laryngopharynx and larynx. Gives instinctive sensation to the heart and stomach viscera.

- Special Sensory: There is a taste sensation that occurs in the epiglottis and foundation of the tongue.

- Motor: Provides engine innervation to most of the muscles of the pharynx, delicate sense of taste, and larynx.

- Parasympathetic: Innervates the smooth muscle of the trachea, bronchi and gastro-intestinal tract, and controls heart mood.

The vagus nerve, when associated to the parasympathetic side, tends to diminish readiness, circulatory strain, and pulse. It also assists with tranquillity, unwinding, and assimilation. Subsequently, the vagus nerve additionally assists with crap, pee, and sexual excitement.

Different vagus nerve impacts include:

- Communication between the cerebrum and the gut: The vagus nerve conveys data from the gut to the mind.

- Relaxation with profound breathing: The vagus nerve speaks with the stomach. With full breaths, an individual feels increasingly loose.

- Decreasing irritation: The vagus nerve sends a mitigating sign to different parts of the body.

- Lowering the pulse and circulatory strain: If the vagus nerve is overactive, it can prompt the heart being not able to siphon enough blood around the body. At times, unnecessary vagus nerve movement can cause loss of awareness and organ harm.

- Fear the executives: The vagus nerve sends data from the gut to the cerebrum, which is connected to managing pressure, tension, and dread - consequently the adage, "hunch." This assists an individual in recouping from distressing and frightening circumstances.

Anatomical (The Course)

Be aware that the vagus nerve has the longest course of all the cranial nerves, reaching out from the head to the guts.

In the Head

The vagus nerve starts from the medulla of the brainstem. It leaves the noggin by means of the jugular foramen, with the glossopharyngeal and embellishment nerves (CN IX and XI individually).

Inside the noggin, the auricular branch emerges. This provides sensation to the back piece of the outer sound-related trench and outside ear.

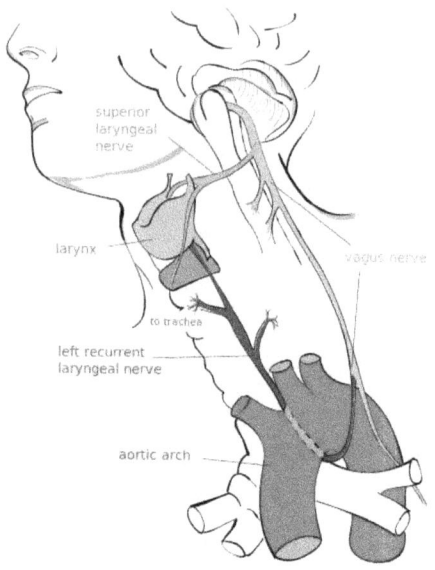

Fig 1.0 – Overview of the major branches of the vagus nerve

In the neck, the vagus nerve goes into the carotid sheath, voyaging poorly with the inside jugular vein and regular carotid corridor. At the base of the neck, the left nerves have varying pathways:

- The right vagus nerve passes foremost to the subclavian supply route and back to the sternoclavicular joint, entering the thorax.

- The left vagus nerve passes poorly between the left basic carotid and left subclavian supply routes, back to the sternoclavicular joint, entering the thorax.

- A few branches emerge in the neck:

- Pharyngeal branches – Provides engine innervation to most of the muscles of the pharynx and delicate sense of taste.

- Superior laryngeal nerve – Splits into inside and outer branches. The outside laryngeal nerve innervates the cricothyroid muscle of the larynx. The inside laryngeal gives tactile innervation to the laryngopharynx and prevalent piece of the larynx.

- Recurrent laryngeal nerve (right side just) – Hooks underneath the subclavian artery supply route, at that point climbs towards to the larynx. It innervates most of the inborn muscles of the larynx.

In the Thorax

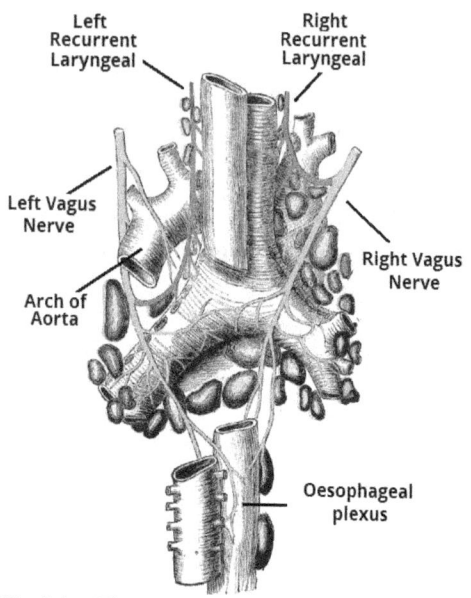

Fig 1.1 – The recurrent laryngeal nerves (The origin)

In the thorax, the correct vagus nerve shapes the back vagal trunk, and the left structures, the front vagal trunk. Branches from the vagal trunks add to the arrangement of the oesophageal plexus, which innervates the smooth muscle of the throat.

Two different branches emerge in the thorax:

- Left intermittent laryngeal nerve – it snares under the curve of the aorta, climbing to innervate most of the natural muscles of the larynx.

- Cardiac branches – these innervate direct pulse and give instinctive sensation to the organ.

- The vagal trunks enter the midriff by means of the oesophageal rest, an opening in the stomach.

In the Abdomen

In the guts, the vagal trunks end by isolating into branches that supply the throat, stomach, and the little and huge gut (up to the splenic flexure).

Tangible Functions

There are substantial and instinctive segments to the tactile capacity of the vagus nerve.

Substantial alludes to sensation from the skin and muscles. This is given by the auricular nerve, which innervates the skin of the back piece of the outside sound-related waterway and outer ear.

The vagus nerve brings about –

- Laryngopharynx – through the inner laryngeal nerve.
- Superior part of larynx (above vocal folds) – through the inner laryngeal nerve.
- Heart – by means of cardiovascular parts of the vagus nerve.
- Up to the splenic flexure (Gastro-intestinal tract) – by means of the terminal parts of the vagus nerve.

Uncommon Sensory Functions

The vagus nerve has a minor job in taste sensation. It conveys afferent filaments from the foundation of the tongue and epiglottis.

(This isn't to be mistaken for the uncommon impression of the glossopharyngeal nerve, which gives taste sensation to the back 1/3 of the tongue).

Engine Functions

The vagus nerve innervates most of the muscles related with the pharynx and larynx. These muscles are answerable for the inception of gulping and phonation.

Pharynx

The greater parts of the muscles of the pharynx are innervated by the pharyngeal parts of the vagus nerve:

- Superior, center, and second-rate pharyngeal constrictor muscles
- Palatopharyngeus
- Salpingopharyngeus

An extra muscle of the pharynx, the stylopharyngeus, is innervated by the glossopharyngeal nerve.

Larynx

Innervation to the natural muscles of the larynx is

accomplished by means of the intermittent laryngeal nerve and outside part of the prevalent laryngeal nerve.

Intermittent laryngeal nerve:

- Thyro-arytenoid
- Posterior crico-arytenoid
- Lateral crico-arytenoid
- Transverse and angled arytenoids
- Vocalis

Outer laryngeal nerve:

- Cricothyroid

Different Muscles

Notwithstanding the pharynx and larynx, the vagus nerve likewise innervates the palatoglossus of the tongue, and most of the muscles of the delicate sense of taste.

Parasympathetic Functions

In the thorax and midriff, the vagus nerve is the fundamental parasympathetic outpouring to the heart and gastro-intestinal organs.

The Heart

Cardiovascular branches emerge in the thorax, passing on parasympathetic innervation to the sino-atrial and atrio-ventricular hubs of the heart. These branches animate a decrease in the resting pulse. They are always dynamic, creating a cadence of 60 – 80 beats for each moment. On the off chance that the vagus nerve was lesioned, the resting pulse would associate with 100 beats for each moment.

Gastro-Intestinal System

The vagus nerve gives parasympathetic innervation to most of the stomach organs. It sends branches to the throat, stomach, and the vast majority of the intestinal tract – up to the splenic flexure of the enormous colon.

The capacity of the vagus nerve is to invigorate smooth muscle withdrawal and glandular emissions in these organs. For instance, in the stomach, the vagus nerve expands the pace of gastric exhausting, and invigorates corrosive creation.

Vagus-Nerve Testing

To test the vagus nerve, a specialist may check the stifler reflex. During this piece of the assessment, the specialist may utilize a delicate cotton swab to tickle the back of the throat on the two sides. This should make the individual stifle. In the event that the individual doesn't choke, this might be because of an issue with the vagus nerve.

Vagus Nerve Issues

Nerve Harm

Mischief to the vagus nerve can have an extent of signs in light of the fact that the nerve is so long and impacts various zones.

The potential signs of mischief to the vagus nerve include:

- difficulty talking or loss of voice
- a voice that is rough or wheezy
- trouble drinking fluids
- loss of the muffle reflex
- pain in the ear
- unusual pulse
- abnormal circulatory strain
- decreased generation of stomach corrosive
- nausea or regurgitating
- abdominal swelling or agony

The manifestation somebody may have depends on what portion of the nerve is harmed.

Gastroparesis

Specialists accept that harm to the vagus nerve may likewise cause a condition called gastroparesis. This condition influences the automatic withdrawals of the stomach-related framework, which keeps the stomach from appropriately purging.

Indications of gastroparesis include:

- nausea or spewing, particularly retching undigested nourishment hours subsequent to eating
- feeling full soon after beginning a feast or total loss of craving
- acid reflux
- abdominal torment or swelling
- unexplained weight reduction
- fluctuations in glucose

A few people create gastroparesis subsequent to experiencing a vagotomy method, which evacuates all or part of the vagus nerve.

Vasovagal syncope

Some of the time, the vagus nerve overcompensates to certain pressure triggers, for example,

- exposure to extraordinary warmth
- fear of real damage
- having blood drawn or the sight of blood
- attempting to have a solid discharge or straining
- standing for quite a while

Keep in mind, the vagus nerve animates certain muscles in the heart that help to slow pulse. At the point when it goes overboard, it can cause an unexpected drop in pulse and circulatory strain, bringing about blacking out. This is known as vasovagal syncope.

Vagus Nerve Incitement

Vagus nerve incitement includes setting a gadget in the body that utilizes electrical driving forces to mimic the nerve. It's utilized to treat a few instances of epilepsy and discouragement that don't react to different medicines.

The gadget is generally put under the skin of the chest, where a wire interfaces it to one side vagus nerve. When the gadget is initiated, it sends flag through the vagus nerve to your brainstem, which at that point transmits data to your mind. A nervous system specialist typically programs the gadget; however, individuals regularly get a handheld magnet they can use to control the gadget all alone also.

This is a significant nerve to each organ it is in contact with. It is the thing that helps control nervousness and sadness in the cerebrum. How we associate with each other is firmly identified with the vagus nerve, as it's joined to nerves that tune our ears to discourse, directs eye to eye connection, and those that control articulations. This nerve likewise has the ability to influence legitimate hormone discharge in the body, which keeps our psychological and physical frameworks sound.

It is the vagus nerve that is liable for expanding

stomach acridity and stomach-related juice discharge for straightforwardness in assimilation in the stomach. At the point when invigorated, it can likewise assist you with absorbing nutrient B12. At the point when it isn't working appropriately, you would then be able to hope to have genuine gut issues, for example, Colitis, IBS, and Re-transition, just to give some examples. Re-transition issues are because of a vagus nerve issue on the grounds that it likewise controls the throat. It's the inappropriate reflex of the throat that causes conditions like Gerd and Re-transition.

The vagus nerve likewise helps control the pulse and circulatory strain, anticipating coronary illness. While in the liver and pancreas, it's this nerve that controls blood glucose balance, averting diabetes. At the point when it goes through the gallbladder, the vagus nerve discharges bile, which is the thing that helps your body in killing poisons and separating fat. While in the bladder, it's this nerve that advances general kidney work, expanding blood stream, accordingly improving filtration in our bodies. At the point when the vagus nerve gets to the spleen, enactment will diminish irritation in all objective organs. This nerve even has the ability to control fruitfulness and climaxes in ladies. An inert or blocked vagus nerve can unleash ruin all through the brain and body.

Since we realize that the vagus nerve is associated with all the significant organs and legitimate working of those organs, we can infer that any turmoil, sickness, or infection of the brain, body, or soul can be turned around or even restored by initiating and animating the vagus nerve. So you will in fact observe beneficial outcomes from vagus nerve incitement on issues, for example, uneasiness issue, coronary illness, cerebral pains and headaches, fibromyalgia, liquor habit, course, gut issues, memory issues, state-of-mind issue, MS, and significantly malignant growth.

There are many archived approaches to invigorate the vagus nerve, for example, singing or reciting, chuckling, yoga, contemplation, breathing activities, practice all in all, and sound just to give some examples. Singing and chuckling works the muscles at the back of your throat, which initiates the nerve. Mellow practicing and practicing expands gut liquids which implies that the vagus nerve has been animated. A controlled Yoga practice can likewise build actuation of this nerve because of the developments, yet in addition the Meditation and OM-ing invigorates the vagus nerve.

Discoveries of full recurrence of organs is going on worldwide by specialists to help in vibrating the body over into a condition of wellbeing, and transfuse sickness and illnesses, for example, nervousness, PTSD, headaches, sadness, memory issues, interminable agony, rest issue, and considerably malignant growth.

"You can truly take a gander at infection as a structure or disharmony," says Dr. Gaynor chief of oncology at the Strang-Cornell Cancer Prevention Center in New York, and creator of Sounds of Healing. "We realize that sound and music effects affect the resistantance framework, which unmistakably have a ton to do with disease."

Sound is quickly getting to be one of the most, to a great extent, hummed about guardians of wellbeing in elective recuperating modalities today! Sound is a splendid execution of basic drug to animate the vagus nerve advancing the wellbeing and essentialness of the considerable number of organs in your body. Do this through sound recuperating and Crystal Chakra Singing Bowls. Clear Quartz is known as the 'Ace Healer' since it can intensify, change, and move vitality. When working with these quartz precious stone dishes, the impacts on the organs, tissues, and cells, alongside the circulatory, endocrine, and metabolic frameworks are serious. The tones from the gems are heard by the ear, felt in the body, and animate the vagus nerve, empowering the vibrations to resound likewise through each Chakra focused in the body, making a reasonable and revived personality, body, and soul!

Epilepsy

In 1997, the FDA permitted the utilization of vagus nerve incitement for hard-headed epilepsy. This includes a little electrical gadget, like a pacemaker, being put in an individual's chest. A slight wire known as a lead keeps running from the gadget to the vagus nerve.

The gadget is put in the body by medical procedure under general soporific. It, at that point, sends electrical driving forces at customary interims, for the duration of the day, to the mind by means of the vagus nerve to decrease the seriousness, or even stop seizures.

Vagus nerve incitement for epilepsy may have some symptoms including sore throat and trouble gulping.

Symptoms of vagus nerve incitement for epilepsy include:

- hoarseness or changes in voice
- sore throat
- shortness of breath
- coughing
- slow pulse
- difficulty gulping
- stomach uneasiness or queasiness

Individuals utilizing this type of treatment ought to consistently tell their primary care physician on the off chance that they are having any issues, as there might be approaches to lessen or stop these.

Entrancing FACTS ABOUT THE VAGUS NERVE

The vagus nerve is so named in light of the fact that it "meanders" like a drifter, conveying tangible filaments from your brainstem to your instinctive organs. The vagus nerve, the longest of the cranial nerves, controls your inward operational hub—the parasympathetic sensory system. Furthermore, it regulates an immense scope of significant capacities, imparting engine and tactile driving forces to each organ in your body. New research has uncovered that it might likewise be the missing connect to treating constant irritation, and the start of an energizing new field of treatment for genuine, serious illnesses.

Here are nine realities about this ground-breaking nerve pack:

1. THE VAGUS NERVE PREVENTS INFLAMMATION.

A specific measure of aggravation after damage or disease is ordinary. In any case, an excess is connected to numerous illnesses and conditions, from sepsis to the immune system condition rheumatoid joint inflammation. The vagus nerve works a tremendous system of filaments positioned like covert agents around the entirety of your organs. At the point when it gets a sign for beginning irritation—the nearness of cytokines or a substance called tumor corruption factor (TNF)— it alarms the mind and draws out mitigating synapses that manage the body's insusceptible reaction.

2. IT HELPS YOU MAKE MEMORIES.

A University of Virginia study in rodents demonstrated that invigorating their vagus nerves reinforced their memory. The activity discharged the synapse norepinephrine into the amygdala, which solidified recollections. Related examinations were done in people, proposing promising medications for conditions like Alzheimer's infection.

3. IT HELPS YOU BREATHE.

The synapse acetylcholine, evoked by the vagus nerve, advises your lungs to relax. It's one reason that Botox—regularly utilized cosmetically—can be possibly perilous, on the grounds that it interferes with your acetylcholine creation. You can, nonetheless, additionally animate your vagus nerve by doing stomach breathing or holding your breath for four to eight checks.

4. IT'S INTIMATELY INVOLVED WITH YOUR HEART.

The vagus nerve is liable for controlling the pulse by means of electrical driving forces to specific muscle tissue—the heart's normal pacemaker—in the correct chamber, where acetylcholine discharges eases back the beat. By estimating the time between your individual heart thumps, and afterward plotting this on a graph over the long run, specialists can decide your pulse changeability, or HRV. This information can offer pieces of information about the flexibility of your heart and vagus nerve.

5. IT INITIATES YOUR BODY'S RELAXATION RESPONSE.

When your ever-careful thoughtful sensory system fires up the battle or flight reactions, pouring the pressure hormone cortisol and adrenaline into your body, the vagus nerve advises your body to relax by discharging acetylcholine. The vagus nerve's ringlets reach out to numerous organs, acting like fiber-optic links that send directions to discharge compounds and proteins like prolactin, vasopressin, and oxytocin, which quiet you down. Individuals with a more grounded vagus reaction might be bound to recuperate all the more rapidly after pressure, damage, or sickness.

6. TRANSLATES BETWEEN YOUR BRAIN OR YOUR GUT.

Your gut utilizes the vagus nerve as a walkie-talkie to tell your mind how you're feeling through electric driving forces called "activity possibilities." Your premonitions are genuine.

7. THE MOST COMMON CAUSE OF FAINTING IS WHEN THERE IS OVERSTIMULATION OF THE VAGUS NERVE.

In the event that you tremble or get squeamish at seeing blood or while getting an influenza shot, you're not powerless. You're encountering "vagal syncope." Your body, reacting to pressure, overstimulates the vagus nerve, causing your circulatory strain and pulse to drop. During outrageous syncope, blood stream is confined to your mind, and you lose cognizance. In any case, more often than not you simply need to sit or rest for the manifestations to die down.

8. THE VAGUS NERVE'S ELECTRICAL STIMULATION REDUCES INFLAMMATION AND MAY INHIBIT IT ALTOGETHER.

Neurosurgeon Kevin Tracey was the first to demonstrate that invigorating the vagus nerve can essentially lessen irritation. Results on rodents were so effective, then he repeated the investigation in people with staggering outcomes. The formation of inserts to animate the vagus nerve by means of electronic inserts demonstrated an extreme decrease, and even reduction, in rheumatoid joint inflammation—which has no known fix and is regularly treated with the lethal medications—hemorrhagic stun, and other similarly genuine incendiary disorders.

9. A NEW FIELD OF MEDICINE HAS BEEN CREATED THROUGH VAGUS NERVE STIMULATION

Prodded on by the accomplishment of vagal nerve incitement to treat irritation and epilepsy, an expanding field of restorative investigation, known as bioelectronics, might be the eventual fate of medication. Utilizing inserts that convey electric driving forces to different body parts, researchers and specialists would like to treat sickness with less drugs and less symptoms.

The vagus nerve manages numerous basic parts of human physiology, including the pulse, circulatory strain, perspiring, assimilation, and in any event, talking. Therefore, restorative science has since quite a while ago looked for methods for balancing the capacity of the vagus nerve.

Life Systems of the Vagus Nerve

The vagus nerve (otherwise called the tenth cranial nerve or CN X) is an exceptionally long nerve that begins in the cerebrum stem and reaches out down through the neck and into the chest and guts. On the off chance, that conveys both engine and tactile data, and it supplies innervation to the heart, significant veins, aviation routes, lungs, throat, stomach, and digestion tracts.

While there are really two vagus nerves (the left and the right), specialists ordinarily allude to them together as "the vagus nerve."

The vagus nerve helps control a few muscles of the throat and of the voice box. It assumes a significant job in controlling the pulse and keeping the gastrointestinal tract in working request. The vagus nerves additionally convey tangible data from the inside organs back to the cerebrum.

Capacity of the Vagus Nerve

Maybe the best hugeness of the vagus nerve is that it is the body's significant parasympathetic nerve, providing parasympathetic strands to all the significant organs of the head, neck, chest, and stomach area. The vagus nerve is answerable for the stifler reflex (and the hack reflex when the ear channel is animated), easing back the pulse, controlling perspiring, managing circulatory strain, invigorating peristalsis of the gastrointestinal tract, and controlling vascular tone.

Kidney and Bladder

The vagus nerve has been demonstrated to advance general kidney work. It expands blood stream and aides in glucose control, which at that point improves blood filtration.

Vagus initiation prompts the arrival of dopamine in kidneys, which discharge sodium and, in this manner, brings down circulatory strain.

A symptom of the vagus nerve is that it causes urinary maintenance as it prompts the bladder. Another approach to see it is that a brought down vagus incitement can make you pee as often as possible.

Mind

For the mind, the vagus nerve helps in temperament and monitors uneasiness and sorrow. The nerve is the one answerable for the mind-body association since it goes out to the majority of the significant organs (except for the adrenal and thyroid organs).

The vagus nerve is personally connected with how we interface with each other, as in, it interfaces legitimately to the nerves that tune our ears to human discourse, manage passionate articulations, and facilitate vision. It is likewise what impacts the arrival of the hormone oxytocin that is significant for social holding.

Studies recommend that a higher vagal tone is generally connected with progressively charitable conduct and more prominent closeness to other people.

The Vasovagal Reflex

Unexpected incitement of a vagus nerve can create what is known as a "vasovagal reflex," which comprises of an abrupt drop in circulatory strain and an easing back of the pulse. This reflex can be activated by gastrointestinal ailment or because of torment, trepidation, or unexpected pressure. A few people are especially inclined to the vasovagal reflex, and their circulatory strain and pulse changes can cause loss of awareness — a condition called "vasovagal syncope."

Over-the-top actuation of the vagus nerve is additionally found in certain ailments, particularly the dysautonomias. Invigorating the vagus nerve can have remedial impacts, (for example, halting scenes of supraventricular tachycardia (SVT) or hiccups), and can help specialists analyze specific sorts of heart mumbles. Vagal incitement can be accomplished effectively by utilizing the Valsalva move.

The Vagus Nerve and the Heart

The correct vagus nerve supplies the sinus hub, and its incitement can deliver sinus bradycardia. The left vagus nerve supplies the AV hub, and its incitement can deliver a type of heart square. It is by creating transient heart obstruct that the Valsalva move can end numerous sorts of SVT.

Gut

In the gut, the vagus nerve expands stomach-related juice emission, stomach sharpness, and gut stream. In the event that there is less vagus incitement, it could expand the danger of IBS, which is the aftereffect of less stream. That is the reason the vagus nerve is significant for expanding gut stream (motility).

Vagus nerve incitement expands the arrival of histamine by stomach cells, which aides in discharging stomach corrosive. Consequently, low stomach acridity is an issue in the vagus nerve.

The vagus nerve is imperative to enable you to retain nutrient B12 by discharging characteristic factor.

After a supper, unwinding and satiety are brought about by enactment of the vagus nerve's transmission to the cerebrum in light of nourishment consumption.

The vagus nerve is pivotal for conditions, for example, GERD in light of the fact that it controls stomach causticity and the throat.

Liver, Pancreas, and Gallbladder

The vagus nerve enables control to blood glucose balance in the liver and pancreas.

For the gallbladder, the vagus nerve helps discharge

bile, which is the thing that disposes of poisons and separates fat.

Heart

In the heart, the vagus nerve controls circulatory strain and pulse.

Animating the vagus nerve anticipates the danger of coronary illness just as other deadly ailments.

Mouth and Ears

The vagus nerve enables control to taste and spit in the tongue and discharges tears in the eyes.

It additionally clarifies why an individual hacks when tickled on their ears, for example, the situation when you're attempting to evacuate ear wax with q-tips or a cotton swab. It can likewise help individuals with tinnitus because of its association with the ear.

Spleen

In the spleen, vagus initiation decreases aggravation by discharging acetylcholine.

Despite the fact that the enactment focuses on the most significant organs, the reaction is more systematic in the spleen.

Since the vagus nerve interfaces with a lady's cervix, uterus, and vagina, it helps control their climaxes and ripeness.

Potential SYMPTOMS OF VAGUS NERVE DYSFUNCTION

- Brain issues
- Obesity and weight gain
- Anxiety
- Depression
- IBS
- High and low pulse
- Chronic exhaustion
- Delayed gastric purging or gastroparesis
- Difficulty in gulping
- B12 insufficiency
- Dizziness/blacking out
- Heartburn
- Chronic irritation

Clutters THAT VAGUS NERVE ACTIVATION CAN FIGHT

Given that the vagus nerve is connected with a wide range of capacities and mind areas, a few kinds of research have revealed the positive advantages of vagal incitement on various infections and conditions, for example,

- OCD
- Alzheimer's

- Migraines
- Heart illness
- Anxiety issue
- Tinnitus
- Obesity
- Fibromyalgia
- Memory issue
- Chronic cardiovascular breakdown
- Multiple sclerosis
- Bulimia
- Autism
- Alcohol enslavement
- Cancer
- Mood issue
- Leaky Gut
- Bad blood flow
- Severe mental infections

The Vagus Nerve in Medical Therapy

Since the vagus nerve has such a large number of significant capacities, medicinal science has been keen, in decades, on utilizing vagus nerve incitement, or vagus nerve obstructing, in restorative treatment.

For a considerable length of time, the vagotomy system (cutting the vagus nerve) was a backbone of treatment for peptic ulcer malady, since this was a method for diminishing the measure of peptic corrosive being delivered by the stomach. Notwithstanding, the vagotomy had a few unfriendly impacts.

Today, there is extraordinary enthusiasm for utilizing electronic triggers (basically, changed pacemakers) to constantly invigorate the vagus nerve trying to treat different therapeutic issues. Such gadgets (alluded to conventionally as vagus nerve invigorating gadgets, or VNS gadgets) have been utilized effectively to treat individuals with extreme epilepsy that is headstrong to sedate treatment. VNS treatment is likewise now and then used to treat unmanageable misery.

Since when you have a sledge everything resembles a nail, organizations that make VNS gadgets are researching their utilization in a few different conditions including hypertension, headaches, tinnitus, fibromyalgia, and weight reduction.

Approaches to Unlock the Powers of the Vagus Nerve

In contrast to different Vegas, what occurs in this vagus doesn't remain there. The vagus nerve is a long wandering heap of engine and tactile strands that connect the mind stem to the heart, lungs, and gut. It additionally branches out to contact and cooperate with the liver, spleen, gallbladder, ureter, female ripeness organs, neck, ears, tongue, and kidneys. It powers up our automatic operational hub—the parasympathetic sensory system— and controls oblivious body capacities, just as everything from keeping our pulse consistent and nourishment assimilation to breathing and perspiring. It likewise directs pulse and blood glucose balance, advances general kidney work, helps discharge bile and testosterone, animates the emission of spit, helps with controlling taste and discharging tears, and assumes a significant job in ripeness issues and climaxes in ladies.

The vagus nerve has filaments that innervate for all intents and purposes the majority of our inward organs. The administration and handling of feelings happens through the vagal nerve between the heart, mind, and gut, which is the reason we have a solid gut response to exceptional mental and enthusiastic states.

Vagus nerve brokenness can bring about an entire host of issues including weight, bradycardia (anomalous moderate heartbeat), trouble gulping, gastrointestinal ailments, swooning, mindset issue, B12 lack, interminable aggravation, hindered hack, and seizures.

This Super Nerve (A Closer Look)

Be aware that just the spinal segment is a bigger nerve framework. Around 80 percent of its nerve strands—or four of its five 'paths'— drive data from the body to the cerebrum. Its fifth path keeps running the other way, moving sign from the cerebrum all through the body. Tied down in the cerebrum stem, the vagus goes through the neck and into the chest, parting into the left vagus and the correct vagus. Every one of these streets is made out of countless nerve filaments that branch into the heart, lungs, stomach, pancreas and about each other organ in the belly.

The vagus nerve utilizes the synapse acetylcholine, which animates muscle compressions in the parasympathetic sensory system. A synapse is a sort of synthetic dispatcher discharged toward the finish of a nerve fiber, that takes into account sign to be moved along from point to point, which animate different organs. For instance, if our mind couldn't speak with our stomach through the arrival of acetylcholine from the vagus nerve, at that point we would quit relaxing.

A few substances, for example, botox and the overwhelming metal mercury, can meddle with acetylcholine creation. Botox has been known to close down the vagus nerve, which causes demise. Mercury obstructs the activity of acetylcholine. At the point when mercury appends to the thiol protein in the heart muscle receptors, the heart muscle can't get the vagus nerve electrical motivation for withdrawal. Cardiovascular issues typically arise. Mercury utilized in fillings just crawls from the cerebrum just as the 3,000 tons of mercury put into the air can meddle with acetylcholine creation. Mercury-loaded immunizations may likewise assume a job in vagus nerve-related chemical imbalance in youngsters.

It's likewise accepted that diet assumes a job in vagus nerve wellbeing. An obesogenic 'cafeteria diet' (high-fat, high-carb lousy nourishment) decreases the affectability of the vagus nerve. Zesty nourishments can likewise make it fizzle.

This is on the grounds that the enteric sensory system (ENS), which oversees the capacity of the gastrointestinal tract, speaks with the focal sensory system (the mind) by means of the vagus nerve. This is known as the gut-cerebrum hub. The ENS is once in a while alluded to as the subsequent cerebrum or reinforcement mind focused in our sunlight based plexus.

The vagus nerve utilizes the synapse acetylcholine, which animates muscle compressions in the parasympathetic sensory system. A synapse is a sort of concoction errand person discharged toward the finish of a nerve fiber that takes into account sign to be moved along from point to point, which invigorate different organs. For instance, if our cerebrum couldn't speak with our stomach by means of the arrival of acetylcholine from the vagus nerve, at that point we would quit relaxing.

The vagus nerve consistently has an effect on everything in individuals with gut issues, nourishment sensitivities, weakness, nervousness, depersonalization, and cerebrum mist. This implies individuals have an ease off vagal volume, i.e., having a lower capacity to play out its capacities.

The one issue to address in this circumstance is to discover which part of the vagus nerve is failing and to what degree it is the issue contrasted with different parts of your science.

Vagus nerve harm can likewise be brought about by diabetes, liquor addiction, upper respiratory viral contaminations, or having some portion of the nerve cut off inadvertently during an activity. Stress can arouse the nerve, alongside exhaustion and uneasiness. In any event, something as basic as awful stance can contrarily affect the vagus nerve.

A Feeling in Your Gut

At the point when individuals state they feel it in their gut, that is not only creative mind, as indicated by Dr. Imprint Sircus, acupuncturist, and specialist of Oriental and peaceful medication.

Our gut impulses are not dreams; however, genuine apprehensive sign that guide quite a bit of our lives.

This is on the grounds that the enteric sensory system (ENS), which oversees the capacity of the gastrointestinal tract, speaks with the focal sensory system (the mind) by means of the vagus nerve. This is known as the gut-cerebrum hub. The ENS is now and then alluded to as the subsequent mind or reinforcement cerebrum focused in our sun based plexus. Sircus proceeds:

"We presently realize that the ENS isn't only fit for self-governance yet in addition impacts the cerebrum. Truth be told, around 90 percent of the sign going along the vagus nerve come not from above, yet from the ENS."

Keeping the gut and vagus nerve passage solid affects our psychological wellness. An ongoing report demonstrates how anti-toxins can make us forceful when they upset the microbiome balance in our gut. A significant examination a year ago by McMaster University in Hamilton, Ontario, Canada, found that specific advantageous gut microorganisms can really counteract PTSD. However, probiotics can help keep vagus nerve flag and the gut in a more beneficial state, as indicated by a report in the National Center for Biotechnology Information (NCBI).

VNS REDUCES ARTHRITIC INFLAMMATION DRAMATICALLY

A joint group of scientists from the United States and Amsterdam led a clinical preliminary and inferred that invigorating the vagus nerve with a little embedded gadget decreased aggravation essentially and improved results for patients with rheumatoid joint inflammation by hindering cytokine generation.

As per scientists, rheumatoid joint inflammation (RA) is a constant incendiary malady that has influenced over 1.3 million individuals in the United States and people spend a huge number of dollars to treat it every year.

For this examination, the neuroscientists and immunology-specialists utilized cutting edge innovation so as to delineate neural hardware that directs irritation.

One circuit, known as the "provocative reflex," shows that there are activity possibilities that are transmitted in the vagus nerve which prevent the generation of cytokines.

This is viewed as the primary human investigation of its sort to diminish rheumatoid joint pain side effects by invigorating the vagus nerve with a little embedded gadget that set off a chain response and subsequently, decreased cytokine levels and aggravation.

What's more, despite the fact that the examination was centered around rheumatoid joint pain, the outcomes likewise gave constructive ramifications to individuals experiencing different infections, including Crohn's, Alzheimer's, and Parkinson's.

Boosting with Electricity

Specialists have since quite a while ago abused the nerve's impact on the cerebrum. Electrical incitement of the vagus nerve, called vagus nerve incitement (VNS), is at times used to treat individuals with epilepsy or melancholy. VNS is intended to anticipate seizures by sending customary, gentle beats of electrical vitality to the cerebrum by means of the vagus nerve. These heartbeats are provided by a gadget, something like a pacemaker. It is put under the skin on the chest divider and a wire keeps running from it to the vagus nerve in the neck. Scientists concentrating the impacts of vagus incitement on epilepsy saw that patients encountered a second advantage random to seizure decrease: their temperaments likewise improved.

According to a report distributed in the (PNAS) also known as Proceedings of the National Academy of Sciences (PNAS), it indicated how invigorating the vagus nerve with a bioelectronic gadget "fundamentally improved proportions of infection action in patients with rheumatoid joint pain," a ceaseless provocative illness that influences 1.3 million individuals in the USA and costs several billions of dollars yearly to treat.

12 Vagus Nerve Stimulation Techniques

The vagus nerve shouldn't be stunned into shape. It can likewise be conditioned and reinforced like a muscle. Here are some basic things you can do that may improve your wellbeing especially:

1. Positive Social Relationships – An investigation had members contemplate others while quietly rehashing positive expressions about loved ones. Contrasted with the controls, the meditators demonstrated a general increment in positive feelings like tranquillity, happiness, and expectation in the wake of finishing the class. These positive musings of others prompted an improvement in vagal capacity as found in pulse changeability. The outcomes additionally demonstrated a more conditioned vagus nerve than when basically ruminating.

2. Cold – "Cold introduction, for example, chilly showers or face dunking invigorates the nerve also," says Mentore.

Studies demonstrate that when your body changes with cold, your battle or flight (thoughtful) framework decays and your rest and condensation (parasympathetic) framework increments and this is intervened by the vagus nerve. Any sort of intense cold introduction including drinking super cold water will build vagus nerve actuation.

3. Washing – Another home solution for an under-invigorated vagus nerve is to swish with water. Swishing really invigorates the muscles of the bed which are terminated by the vagus nerve.

"Ordinarily patients will tear up a piece which is a decent sign and on the off chance that they don't, we suggest that they do it consistently until they see that they do fire destroying a piece," says Hoffman. "This has been appeared to quickly improve working memory execution."

4. Singing and Chanting – Humming, mantra reciting, psalm singing, and playful enthusiastic singing all expand pulse changeability (HRV) in marginally various ways. Basically, singing resembles starting a vagal siphon conveying loosening up waves. Singing as loud as possible works the muscles in the back of the throat to enact the vagus. Singing as one, which is regularly done in houses of worship and synagogues, likewise builds HRV and vagus work. Singing has been found to expand oxytocin, otherwise called the affection hormone since it makes individuals feel more like each other.

5. Back Rub – You can invigorate your vagus nerve by rubbing your feet and your neck along the carotid sinus, situated along the carotid supply routes on either side of your neck. A neck back rub can help diminish seizures. A foot back rub can help bring down your pulse and circulatory strain. A weight back rub can likewise enact the vagus nerve. These back rubs are utilized to enable newborn children to put on weight by animating gut work.

6. Chuckling – Happiness and giggling are common invulnerable sponsors. Giggling likewise animates the vagus nerve. Research demonstrates how chuckling expands HRV in a gathering domain.

There are different case reports of individuals blacking out from chuckling and this might be from the vagus nerve/parasympathetic framework being animated excessively. Swooning can come after giggling just as pee, hacking, gulping or solid discharge—which are all aided along by vagus initiation.

7. Yoga and Tai Chi — Both increment vagus nerve action and your parasympathetic framework when all is said and done. Studies have demonstrated that yoga expands GABA, a quieting synapse in your cerebrum. Scientists trust it does this by "invigorating vagal afferents (strands)," which increment action in the parasympathetic sensory system. This is particularly useful for the individuals who battle with uneasiness or sadness.

Studies demonstrate that jujitsu likewise can

'upgrade vagal tweak.'

8. Breathing Slowly and Deeply — Every human heart and the neck contains neurons that have receptors also known as baroreceptors, which identify circulatory strain and transmit the neuronal sign to your cerebrum. This enacts your vagus nerve that associates with your heart to lower circulatory strain and pulse. Slow breathing, with a generally equivalent measure of time taking in and out, expands the affectability of baroreceptors and vagal enactment. Breathing around 5-6 breaths for each moment in the normal grown-up can be extremely useful.

9. Exercise – Exercise expands your mind's development hormone, bolsters your cerebrum's mitochondria, and helps turn around psychological decrease. But at the same time it's been known to invigorate the vagus nerve, which prompts valuable cerebrum and emotional well-being impacts. Mellow exercise additionally invigorates gut stream, which is interceded by the vagus nerve.

10. Espresso Enemas — Enemas resemble runs for your vagus nerve. Extending the entrails expands vagus nerve initiation, as is finished with douches. This purging is practiced by expanding the liver's ability to detoxify poisons in the blood and restricting them to the bile. All the while, the liver purges itself as it discharges the lethal bile into the little, at that point huge, digestive tract for clearing. The whole blood supply circles through the liver at regular intervals. By holding the espresso 12 to 15 minutes, the blood will circle four to multiple times

for purging, much like a dialysis treatment. The water substance of the espresso invigorates intestinal peristalsis and purges the internal organ with the collected lethal bile.

11. Nervana — This wearable item sends a delicate electrical wave through the left ear waterway to animate the body's vagus nerve, while matching up with music, which thusly invigorates the arrival of synapses in the cerebrum that produce a quieting sensation all through the body.

12. Unwind – Learning how to chill might be the number one thing to help keep your vagus nerve conditioned.

CHAPTER TWO

VAGUS NERVE: ITS IMPORTANCE TO

WEIGHT LOSS AND HEALTH

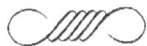

Have you, at any point, asked why a few people feel full in the wake of eating a limited quantity of nourishment and other individuals are as yet hungry until they eat a major serving?

The appropriate response may be in the affectability of their vagus nerve. The vagus nerve is the nerve that associates your gut to your mind, and it's a significant piece of the parasympathetic sensory system (the "rest and summary" reaction, essentially something contrary to "battle or flight").

- All signals going up from the gut to the mind through the vagus nerve influence your possibility of totality or more cravings, your disposition and feelings of anxiety, and the initiation of your provocative pressure reaction.

- Signals running down the vagus nerve from the

cerebrum to the gut influence assimilation, discharge of stomach-related compounds, and gastrointestinal motility (that is an extravagant word for where you are on the scale from clogging to looseness of the bowels).

It's an extremely significant pathway, and vagus nerve initiation is associated with stoutness, gastrointestinal illnesses, cardiovascular sicknesses, disposition issue like despondency, and a wide range of other incessant medical issues.

Here's a glance at why the vagus nerve is so significant, and how your eating routine can improve your wellbeing by influencing vagal nerve signals from the gut.

The Vagus Nerve and Hunger

- The physical greater part of nourishment in the stomach sends satiety flag up the vagus nerve to your mind. This is the manner by which your mind knows to quit feeling hungry after a supper.

- Nutrient detecting and synapses delivered in the gut, similar to serotonin and ghrelin, can likewise send yearning and totality flag up the vagus nerve to the cerebrum.

Corpulence is related with a lower affectability of the vagus nerve to completion signals, and there's a great deal of proof this is caused explicitly by eating routine. Heftiness inciting diets can really adjust the affectability of the vagus nerve to completion signals, so it takes more nourishment for your cerebrum to get the "full presently" signal. Also, much the same as you may expect, invigorating the vagus nerve (to "increase the volume" on the satiety signal) will in general reason weight reduction in test creatures – despite the fact that it's significant that reviews in people have blended outcomes.

The Vagus Nerve and Other Health Issues

Appetite is one integral motivation behind why the vagus nerve is significant. However, in the event that you bring a jump into PubMed, you'll see that vagus nerve brokenness is really connected with a wide range of different issues. That is on the grounds that the vagus nerve likewise manages irritation, and aggravation is engaged with pretty much every ceaseless malady. Invigorating vagus nerve sign to the cerebrum is calming – it flags the mind to turn down the pressure reaction and lessen the generation of incendiary cytokines.

The impacts here are somewhat difficult to unravel in light of the fact that the vagus nerve is a two-way road and there are a ton of convoluted input circles between the cerebrum and the gut (recall that the vagus nerve runs the two different ways!). Be that as it may, for individuals who simply care about improving their wellbeing, the accurate system may be less significant than the outcomes, which are certainly noteworthy:

- Vagus nerve control of irritation influences cardiovascular wellbeing, and vagus nerve incitement may help counteract cardiovascular occasions.

- Vagus nerve flagging is lost in patients with Crohn's Disease (a type of Inflammatory Bowel Disease), and one little, starter concentrate found that vagal nerve incitement helps treat the indications.

- The vagus nerve may likewise be engaged with Irritable Bowel Syndrome, and vagal incitement may be useful for diminishing IBS torment.

- This study is truly intriguing: treating diabetes-inclined rodents with vagal nerve incitement forestalls both sorrow and insulin obstruction.

On the off chance that a terrible eating routine is influencing the effectiveness of your vagus nerve, it could likewise affect every one of these ailments. This could be one motivation behind why gut wellbeing is such a major player in generally speaking wellbeing.

Care and Feeding of Your Vagus Nerve

Up until now, we realize that an obesogenic "cafeteria diet" (high-fat, high-carb shoddy nourishment) diminishes the affectability of the vagus nerve, and that vagus nerve incitement neutralizes that, with enormous advantages for weight... and for pretty much everything else. Lamentably, the "vagal nerve incitement" in these examinations isn't something you can do at home; it's a gadget that the subjects got carefully embedded in their bodies.

However, on the off chance that a lousy eating

routine can lessen the effectiveness of the vagus nerve, possibly a decent diet can help re-establish it. Other than "don't eat a low quality nourishment diet," here's somewhat progressively explicit research.

This examination found that dietary fat decreased aggravation through its impacts on the vagus nerve. The creators inferred that "high-fat… sustenance is possibly remedial in different fiery issue, for example, sepsis and provocative gut infection (IBD) portrayed by an incendiary reaction in which… intestinal obstruction capacity is disabled."

That is upheld up by the association between a ketogenic (exceptionally high-fat, low-carb) diet and vagal nerve incitement as two viable treatments for treatment-safe epilepsy. It's conceivable that a ketogenic diet has a portion of its craving stifling, calming impacts through invigorating the vagus nerve.

This investigation additionally found that a probiotic (Lactobacillus casei strain Shirota) actuated the vagus nerve. The probiotic changed the gut-to-cerebrum stress motioning in understudies taking a distressing test and stifled the arrival of the pressure hormone cortisol.

High-impact exercise may likewise be useful.

For moment satisfaction, you can likewise do your very own vagal nerve incitement utilizing the Valsalva move. Plunk down, in light of the fact that it can make you somewhat dazed. Take a full breath, and afterward close your mouth and squeeze your nose shut with the goal that no air can get away. At that point imagine like you're attempting to inhale out, yet without opening your nose or mouth – you should feel the weight from the air.

Continue doing this for 15-20 seconds, and afterward let the let some circulation into and inhale typically. (On the off chance that you do any weightlifting, this is the kind of breath-holding you do to settle your spine during overwhelming squats and deadlifts.)

The Valsalva move doesn't have long haul impacts; however, it may be useful for a prompt circumstance, similar to directly before a test or in an unpleasant drive.

That is not a great deal to go on – there simply aren't numerous investigations on eating regimen and the vagus nerve. In any case, it's something to begin with, and it backs up the significant ways that the gut, the mind, and the remainder of your body are altogether associated. Thinking about the vagus nerve clarifies why gut wellbeing, psychological wellness, and entire body wellbeing are so tangled up with one another.

CHAPTER THREE

THE ROLE OF THE VAGUS NERVE IN

DEPRESSION

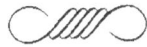

The etiopathogenesis of misery is a profoundly perplexing procedure portrayed by a few neurobiological adjustments incorporating diminished monoamine neurotransmission in the cerebrum, dysregulated hypothalamic-pituitary-adrenal hub action, diminished neuronal versatility, and incessant aggravation in the mind and fringe tissues. Trial and clinical examinations show that the vagus nerve may impact these procedures. The significance of the vagus nerve in the etiopathogenesis of wretchedness is additionally bolstered by its association in the enlistment of affliction conduct, just as by clinical examinations affirming a valuable impact of vagus nerve incitement in discouraged patients. The point of this article is to portray current information of afferent and efferent vagal pathways job in the improvement and movement of despondency.

For reasons that specialists don't totally comprehend, these electrical driving forces transmitted by means of the vagus nerve to the cerebrum can assuage the indications of discouragement. The driving forces may influence the way nerve cell circuits transmit flag in territories of the cerebrum that influence temperament. Nonetheless, it more often than not takes a while before you feel the impacts.

At whatever point it's fundamental, your primary care physician can change the settings on the gadget (basically changing the portion) in the workplace with a programming wand. Ordinarily, the gadget is set to go off at normal interims. You can likewise turn it off utilizing an extraordinary magnet.

Vagus nerve incitement includes the utilization of a gadget to invigorate the vagus nerve with electrical driving forces. An implantable vagus nerve trigger is as of now FDA-affirmed to treat epilepsy and despondency.

In ordinary vagus nerve incitement, a gadget is carefully embedded under the skin on your chest, and a wire is strung under your skin interfacing the gadget to one side vagus nerve. At the point when initiated, the gadget sends electrical flag along the left vagus nerve to your brainstem, which at that point sends sign to specific regions in your mind. The correct vagus nerve isn't utilized in light of the fact that it's bound to convey strands that supply nerves to the heart.

New, noninvasive vagus nerve incitement gadgets, which don't require careful implantation, have been affirmed in Europe to treat epilepsy, wretchedness, and agony. A non-invasive gadget that animates the vagus nerve was as of late endorsed by the Food and Drug Administration for the treatment of bunch cerebral pains in the United States.

Vagus Nerve Incitement

Around 33% of individuals with epilepsy don't completely react to hostile seizure drugs. Vagus nerve incitement might be an alternative to decrease the recurrence of seizures in individuals who haven't accomplished control with prescriptions.

Vagus nerve incitement may likewise be useful for individuals who haven't reacted to concentrated despondency medicines, for example, upper meds, mental guiding (psychotherapy) and electroconvulsive treatment (ECT).

The Food and Drug Administration (FDA) has affirmed vagus nerve incitement for individuals who:

- Are 4 years of age and more established
- Have central (halfway) epilepsy
- Have seizures that aren't well-controlled with prescriptions

The FDA has additionally affirmed vagus nerve incitement for the treatment of melancholy in grown-ups who:

- Have incessant, difficult to-treat despondency (treatment-safe melancholy)

- Haven't improved in the wake of at least four drugs or electroconvulsive treatment (ECT), or both

- Continue standard sorrow medications alongside vagus nerve incitement

Also, analysts are contemplating vagus nerve incitement as a potential treatment for an assortment of conditions, including migraines, rheumatoid joint inflammation, fiery inside ailment, bipolar issue, stoutness and Alzheimer's ailment.

Dangers

For the vast majority, vagus nerve incitement is protected. In any case, it has a few dangers, both from the medical procedure to embed the gadget and from the mind incitement.

Medical procedure dangers

Careful difficulties with embedded vagus nerve incitement are uncommon and are like the perils of having different kinds of medical procedure. They include:

- Pain where the cut (entry point) is made to embed the gadget

- Infection

- Difficulty gulping

- Vocal line loss of motion, which is generally transitory, however can be lasting

Reactions After Medical Procedure

A portion of the reactions and medical issues related with embedded vagus nerve incitement can include:

- Voice changes
- Hoarseness
- Throat torment
- Cough
- Headaches
- Shortness of breath
- Difficulty gulping
- Tingling or prickling of the skin
- Insomnia
- Worsening of rest apnea

For a great many people, reactions are mediocre. They may decrease after some time, yet some symptoms may stay annoying for whatever length of time that you utilize embedded vagus nerve incitement.

Changing the electrical driving forces can help limit these impacts. In the event that reactions are terrible, the gadget can be stopped briefly or for all time.

How You Get Ready

It's critical to painstakingly consider the advantages and disadvantages of embedded vagus nerve incitement before choosing to have the methodology. Ensure you recognize what the majority of your other treatment decisions are and that you and your primary care physician both feel that embedded vagus nerve incitement is the best alternative for you. Ask your primary care physician precisely what you ought to expect during medical procedure and after the beat generator is set up.

Nourishment and Prescriptions

You may need to quit taking certain prescriptions early, and your PCP may ask you not to eat the night prior to the methodology.

What You Can Anticipate Prior to the Methodology

Prior to medical procedure, your primary care physician will do a physical assessment. You may need blood tests or different tests to ensure you don't have any wellbeing worries that may be an issue. Your PCP may have you start taking anti-microbials before medical procedure to forestall contamination.

During the Strategy

Medical procedure to embed the vagus nerve incitement gadget should be possible on an outpatient premise; however, a few specialists suggest remaining medium-term.

The medical procedure, as a rule, takes an hour to 90 minutes. You may stay alert, however have drug to numb the medical procedure zone (nearby anesthesia), or you might be oblivious during the medical procedure (general anesthesia).

The medical procedure itself doesn't include your cerebrum. Two entry points are made: one on your chest or in the armpit (axillary) locale, and the other on the left half of the neck.

The beat generator is embedded in the upper left half of your chest. The gadget is intended to be a perpetual embed, yet it tends to be expelled if vital.

After the Technique

The beat generator is turned on during a visit to your primary care physician's office half a month after medical procedure. At that point, it very well may be customized to convey electrical motivations to the vagus nerve at different terms, frequencies, and flows. Vagus nerve incitement typically begins at a low level and is step by step expanded, contingent upon your indications and symptoms.

Incitement is modified to turn on and off in explicit cycles —, for example, 30 seconds on, five minutes off. You may make them shiver sensations or slight genuine annoyance and transitory raspiness when the nerve incitement is on.

The trigger doesn't distinguish seizure action or melancholy side effects. At the point when it's turned on, the trigger turns on and off at the interims chosen by your primary care physician. You can utilize a hand-held magnet to start incitement at an alternate time, for instance, on the off chance that you sense an approaching seizure.

The magnet can likewise be utilized to incidentally mood-kill the vagus nerve incitement, which might be essential when you do certain exercises, for example, open talking, singing or working out, or when you're eating on the off chance that you have gulping issues.

You'll have to visit your primary care physician occasionally to ensure that the beat generator is working accurately and that it hasn't moved out of position. Check with your PCP before having any medicinal tests, for example, attractive reverberation imaging (MRI), which may meddle with your gadget.

Results

Embedded vagus nerve incitement isn't a solution for epilepsy. The vast majority with epilepsy won't quit having seizures or taking epilepsy drug through and through after the method. Yet, many will have less seizures, up to 20 to 50 percent less. Seizure force may reduce too.

Vagus nerve incitement may likewise abbreviate the recuperation time after a seizure. Individuals who've had vagus nerve incitement to treat epilepsy may likewise encounter enhancements in state of mind and personal satisfaction.

Research is as yet blended on the advantages of

embedded vagus nerve incitement for the treatment of misery. A few investigations recommend the advantages of vagus nerve incitement for wretchedness gather after some time, and it might take at any rate a while of treatment before you see any upgrades in your downturn side effects. Embedded vagus nerve incitement doesn't work for everyone, and it isn't proposed to supplant conventional medications. Moreover, some medical coverage bearers may not pay for this strategy.

Investigations of embedded vagus nerve incitement as a treatment for conditions, for example, Alzheimer's infection, cerebral pains, and rheumatoid joint inflammation have been too little to even think about drawing any authoritative decisions about how well it might function for those issues. More research is required.

CHAPTER FOUR

DISEASES ASSOCIATED WITH THE VAGUS

NERVE AND HOW TO PREVENT THEM

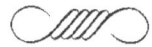

Gastroparesis

Gastroparesis is a condition that influences the typical unconstrained development of the muscles (motility) in your stomach. Conventionally, solid strong compressions impel nourishment through your stomach related tract. Be that as it may, in the event that you have gastroparesis, your stomach's motility is backed off or doesn't work by any means, keeping it from discharging appropriately.

Certain prescriptions, for example, narcotic torment relievers, a few antidepressants, and hypertension and hypersensitivity drugs, can prompt moderate gastric exhausting and cause comparable side effects. For individuals who as of now have gastroparesis, these prescriptions may exacerbate their condition.

Gastroparesis can meddle with typical assimilation, cause sickness and retching, and cause issues with glucose levels and sustenance. The reason for gastroparesis is typically obscure. Once in a while it's an entanglement of diabetes, and a few people create gastroparesis after medical procedure. Despite the fact that there's no remedy for gastroparesis, changes to your eating regimen, alongside drug, can offer some help.

Side Effects

Signs and side effects of gastroparesis include:

- Vomiting
- Nausea
- Vomiting undigested nourishment eaten a couple of hours sooner
- Acid reflux
- Abdominal swelling
- Abdominal torment
- Changes in glucose levels
- Lack of craving
- Weight misfortune and unhealthiness

Numerous individuals with gastroparesis don't have any recognizable signs and side effects.

Causes

It's not in every case clear what prompts gastroparesis. Yet, much of the time, gastroparesis is accepted to be brought about by harm to a nerve that controls the stomach muscles (vagus nerve).

The vagus nerve deals with the intricate procedures in your stomach-related tract, incorporating flagging the muscles in your stomach to agreement and push nourishment into the small digestive tract. A harmed vagus nerve can't send flag typically to your stomach muscles. This may make nourishment stay in your stomach longer, instead of move regularly into your small digestive system to be processed.

The vagus nerve can be harmed by sicknesses, for example, diabetes, or by medical procedure to the stomach or small digestive system.

Hazard Factors

Components that can build your danger of gastroparesis:

- Diabetes

- Abdominal or esophageal medical procedure

- Infection, generally an infection

- Certain meds that moderate the pace of stomach discharging, for example, opiate torment meds

- Scleroderma (a connective tissue ailment)

- Nervous framework ailments, for example, Parkinson's ailment or various sclerosis

- Hypothyroidism (low thyroid)

Ladies are bound to create gastroparesis than men.

Difficulties

Gastroparesis can cause a few difficulties, for example,

- Severe lack of hydration. Continuous spewing can cause lack of hydration.

- Malnutrition. Poor hunger can mean you don't take in enough calories, or you might be not be able assimilate enough supplements because of regurgitating.

- Undigested nourishment that solidifies and stays in your stomach. Undigested nourishment in your stomach can solidify into a strong mass called a bezoar. Bezoars can cause queasiness and spewing and might be dangerous in the event that they keep nourishment from going into your small digestive system.

- Unpredictable glucose changes. In spite of the fact that gastroparesis doesn't cause diabetes, periodic changes in the rate and measure of nourishment going into the little entrails can cause inconsistent changes in glucose levels. These varieties in glucose exacerbate diabetes. Thus, poor control of glucose levels exacerbates gastroparesis.

- Decreased personal satisfaction. An intense erupt of side effects can make it hard to work and stay aware of different duties.

Seizure Disorders

In seizure issue, the cerebrum's electrical action is

occasionally upset, bringing about some level of brief mind brokenness.

- Many individuals have uncommon sensations just before a seizure begins.

- Some seizures cause wild shaking and loss of awareness; however, more regularly, individuals essentially quit moving or become ignorant of what's going on.

- Doctors suspect the conclusion dependent on indications, yet imaging of the mind, blood tests, and electroencephalography (to record the cerebrum's electrical action) are generally expected to recognize the reason.

- If required, medications can, for the most part, help avert seizures.

Ordinary mind capacity requires a deliberate, composed, facilitated release of electrical driving forces. Electrical motivations empower the mind to speak with the spinal line, nerves, and muscles just as inside itself. Seizures may result when the cerebrum's electrical action is disturbed.

About 2% of grown-ups have a seizure eventually during their life. 66% of these individuals never have another. Seizure issue usually start in early adolescence or in late adulthood.

Kinds of Seizures

Seizures might be depicted as pursues:

- Epileptic: These seizures have no clear trigger (that is, they are ridiculous), and they happen at least multiple times. One seizure isn't viewed as epilepsy. Epileptic seizures are known as a seizure issue or epilepsy. What causes epileptic seizures is regularly obscure (called idiopathic epilepsy). Be that as it may, they might be brought about by different cerebrum issue, for example, auxiliary anomalies, strokes, or tumors. In such cases, they are called symptomatic epilepsy. Symptomatic epilepsy is most regular among infants and more seasoned individuals.

- Non-epileptic: These seizures are activated (incited) by a reversible issue or a condition that disturbs the cerebrum, for example, a contamination, a stroke, head damage, or a response to a medication. In youngsters, a fever can trigger a non-epileptic seizure (called a febrile seizure).

Causes

The causes usually depend on when seizures start:

- Before age 2: High fevers or transitory metabolic variations from the norm, for example, unusual blood levels of sugar (glucose), calcium, magnesium, nutrient B6, or sodium, can trigger at least one seizures. Seizures don't happen once the fever or variation from the norm settle. On the off chance that the seizures repeat without such triggers, the reason is probably going to be damage during birth, a birth imperfection, or an inherited metabolic variation from the norm or mind issue.

- 2 to 14 years: Often, the reason is obscure.

- Adults: Head damage, stroke, or tumor may harm the mind, causing a seizure. Liquor withdrawal (brought about by abruptly halting drinking) is a typical reason for seizures.

- Older grown-ups: The reason might be a cerebrum tumor or stroke.

Seizures with no recognizable reason are called idiopathic.

Conditions that aggravate the cerebrum, for example, wounds, certain medications, lack of sleep, contaminations, fever—or that deny the mind of oxygen or fuel, for example, unusual heart rhythms, a low degree of oxygen in the blood, or an extremely low degree of sugar in the blood (hypoglycemia)— can trigger a solitary seizure whether an individual has a seizure issue or not. A seizure that comes from such an upgrade is known as an incited seizure (and in this manner is a non-epileptic seizure).

Individuals with a seizure issue are bound to have a seizure when the following happen:

- They are under abundance physical or passionate pressure.

- They are inebriated or denied of rest.

- They have all of a sudden quit drinking or using tranquilizers.

Maintaining a strategic distance from these conditions can help avert seizures.

Seldom, seizures are activated by tedious sounds, blazing lights, computer games, or in any event, contacting certain pieces of the body. In such cases, the turmoil is called reflex epilepsy.

Manifestations

A quality (bizarre sensations) depicts how an individual feels before a seizure starts, or it might be a piece of a central mindful seizure that is simply beginning. An air may incorporate any of he following:

- Abnormal scents or tastes

- Butterflies in the stomach

- Feeling as though something has been experienced before despite the fact that it has not (called this feels familiar) or the contrary inclination—something appears to be new despite the fact that it is commonplace here and there (called jamais vu)

- An extraordinary inclination that a seizure is going to start.

- Practically all seizures are moderately concise, enduring from a couple of moments to a couple of minutes. Most seizures last 1 to 2 minutes.

Every so often, seizures repeat over and again, as happens in status epilepticus.

The vast majority who have a seizure issue look and

act regularly between seizures.

Side effects of seizures differ contingent upon which zone of the mind is influenced by the strange electrical release, as in the following:

- An strongly lovely or upsetting taste if the piece of the cerebrum called the insula is influenced

- Visual mind flights (seeing unformed pictures) if the occipital flap is influenced

- Inability to talk if the territory that controls discourse (situated in the frontal flap) is influenced

- A seizure (snapping and fits of muscles all through the body) if huge territories on the two sides of the mind are influenced

- Seizures might be delegated

- Motor: Involving anomalous muscle compressions, (for example, jolting of an appendage or seizures)

- Non-motor: Not including anomalous muscle compressions

Other potential indications incorporate deadness or shivering in a particular body part, brief scenes of lethargy, loss of awareness, and disarray. Individuals may upchuck on the off chance that they lose awareness. Individuals may lose control of their muscles, bladder, or guts. A few people keep quiet.

Side effects additionally differ contingent upon whether the seizure is:

- Focal-beginning (the seizure starts in a single side of the mind)
- Generalized-beginning (the seizure starts in the two sides of the mind)

There are a few sorts of central and summed-up seizures. The vast majority have just one sort of seizure. Others have at least two sorts.

A few kinds of seizures might be central or summed up:

- Atonic (including loss of muscle tone)
- Clonic (including cadenced snapping of muscles)
- Tonic (including hardening of muscles)
- Myoclonic (including abrupt, lightning-like snapping of muscles)
- Epileptic (juvenile) fits and febrile seizures, which happen in kids

Central Beginning Seizures

In central beginning seizures, the seizures start in one side of the cerebrum. These seizures are ordered dependent on whether the individual knows during the seizure:

- • Awareness is kept up (called central mindful seizures).
- • Awareness is disabled (called central debilitated mindfulness seizures).

Mindfulness alludes to learning of self and

condition. On the off chance that mindfulness is weakened during any piece of the seizure, the seizure is viewed as a central hindered mindfulness seizure. Specialists decide if individuals stayed mindful during a seizure by asking them or, if a seizure is happening, checking whether they react when addressed.

In central mindful seizures, strange electrical releases start in a little zone of the cerebrum and stay limited to that zone. Since just a little zone of the mind is influenced, side effects are identified with the capacity constrained by that territory. For instance, if the little region of the cerebrum that controls the correct arm's developments (in the left frontal projection) is influenced, the correct arm may automatically be lifted up and snap, and the head may move in the direction of the lifted arm. Individuals are totally cognizant and mindful of the environment. A central mindful seizure may advance to a central debilitated mindfulness seizure.

Jacksonian seizures are a kind of central mindful seizures. Side effects start in one hand or foot, and at that point climb the appendage as the electrical action spreads in the cerebrum. Individuals are totally mindful of what is happening during the seizure.

Other central mindful seizures influence the face, and at that point spread to an arm or now and again a leg.

In central impeded mindfulness seizures, unusual electrical releases start in a little territory of the worldly flap or frontal projection and immediately spread to other close-by zones. The seizures start with an air, which keeps going 1 to 2 minutes. During the atmosphere, individuals begin to put some distance between the environment.

During the seizure, mindfulness winds up disabled; however, individuals don't end up oblivious. Individuals may do the following:

- Stare
- Chew or smack the lips automatically
- Move the hands, arms, and legs in abnormal, purposeless ways
- Utter useless sounds
- Not comprehend what other individuals are stating
- Resist help

A few people can chat; however, their discussion needs immediacy, and the substance is, to some degree, scanty. They might be confounded and muddled. This state may keep going for a few minutes. Every so often, individuals lash out in the event that they are limited.

A few people at that point recuperate completely. In others, the strange electrical release spreads to contiguous territories and to the opposite side of the mind, bringing about a summed-up seizure. Summed-up seizures that result from central seizures are called central to two-sided seizures. That is, they start in one side of the mind and spread to the two sides.

Epilepsia partialis continua is uncommon. Central

seizures happen at regular intervals or minutes for quite a long time to years one after another. They commonly influence an arm, a hand, or one side of the face. These seizures result from:

- In grown-ups: Localized cerebrum harm, (for example, scarring because of a stroke)

- In youngsters: Inflammation of the mind (as happens in encephalitis and measles)

Summed-Up Beginning Seizures

In summed-up beginning seizures, the seizure starts in the two sides of the cerebrum. Most summed-up beginning seizures disable mindfulness. They frequently cause loss of awareness and anomalous developments, normally right away. Loss of cognizance might be brief or keep going quite a while.

Summed-up beginning seizures incorporate the following sorts:

- Tonic-clonic seizures (some time ago, called fabulous mal seizures)

- Clonic seizures

- Tonic seizures

- Atonic seizures

- Myoclonic seizures, including adolescent myoclonic epilepsy

- Epileptic (juvenile) fits

- Absence seizures

Most kinds of summed-up seizures, (for example, tonic-clonic seizures) include strange muscle withdrawals. Those that don't are called nonattendance seizures.

In summed-up tonic-clonic seizures, muscles contract (the tonic part), and at that point quickly shift back and forth among contracting and unwinding (the clonic part). These seizures might be:

- Generalized (beginning in the two sides of the mind)
- Focal to two-sided (beginning in one side of the mind and spreading to the two sides)

In the two sorts, awareness is incidentally lost and a seizure happens when the unusual releases spread to the two sides of the mind.

Summed-up beginning seizures start with irregular releases in a profound, focal piece of the mind and spread all the while to the two sides of the cerebrum. There is no emanation. The seizure regularly starts with a clamor. Individuals at that point become uninformed or lose awareness.

During summed-up beginning seizures, individuals may do the following:

- Have serious muscle fits and yanking all through the body
- Fall down
- Clench their teeth

- Bite their tongue (regularly happens)
- Drool or foam at the mouth
- Lose control of the bladder and additionally entrails

The seizures generally last 1 to 2 minutes. A short time later, a few people, who have a cerebral pain, are incidentally confounded and feel very drained. These indications may last from minutes to hours. A great many people don't recollect what occurred during the seizure.

Central to-reciprocal tonic-clonic (fabulous mal) seizures for the most part start with an unusual electrical release in a little zone of one side of the cerebrum, bringing about a central mindful or central weakened mindfulness seizure. The release at that point rapidly spreads to the two sides of the mind, making the whole cerebrum glitch. Indications are like those of summed-up beginning seizures.

Atonic seizures happen fundamentally in youngsters. They are described by a brief, however complete loss of muscle tone and awareness. They cause kids to tumble to the ground, some of the time bringing about damage.

In clonic seizures, the appendages on the two sides of the body and frequently head, neck, face, and trunk snap musically all through the seizure. Clonic seizures more often than not happen in newborn children. They are considerably less basic than tonic-clonic seizures.

Tonic seizures happen regularly during rest, typically in kids. Muscle tone increments unexpectedly or step by step, making muscles harden. The appendages and neck are regularly influenced. Tonic seizures commonly last just 10 to 15 seconds, however can cause individuals, if remaining, to tumble to the ground. The vast majority don't lose awareness. On the off chance that seizures last more, muscles may twitch a couple of times as the seizure closes.

Atypical nonattendance seizures, atonic seizures, and tonic seizures typically happen as a major aspect of a serious type of epilepsy called Lennox-Gastaut disorder, which starts before kids are 4 years of age.

Myoclonic seizures are described by one or a few appendages or the storage compartment. The seizures are brief and don't cause loss of cognizance; however, they may happen drearily and may advance to a tonic-clonic seizure with loss of awareness.

Adolescent myoclonic epilepsy commonly starts during immaturity. Regularly, seizures start with brisk rascals of the two arms. About 90% of these seizures are trailed by tonic-clonic seizures. A few people additionally have nonattendance seizures. The seizures frequently happen when individuals stir toward the beginning of the day, particularly on the off chance that they are restless. Drinking liquor additionally makes these seizures more probable.

Nonappearance seizures don't include irregular muscle compression. They might be delegated

- Typical (petit mal)

- Atypical

Common nonattendance seizures for the most part start in adolescence, more often than not between the ages of 5 and 15 years, and don't proceed into adulthood. In any case, grown-ups once in a while have commonplace nonappearance seizures. Dissimilar to tonic-clonic seizures, nonattendance seizures don't cause spasms or other sensational side effects. Individuals don't tumble down, break down, or move jerkily. Rather, they have scenes of gazing with rippling eyelids and here and there jerking facial muscles. They ordinarily lose cognizance, winding up totally unconscious of their environment. These scenes last 10 to 30 seconds. Individuals unexpectedly stop what they are doing and continue it similarly as suddenly. They experience no eventual outcomes and don't have a clue that a seizure has happened. Without treatment, numerous individuals have a few seizures every day. Seizures regularly happen when individuals are sitting discreetly. Seizures seldom happen during activity. Hyperventilation can trigger a seizure.

Atypical nonappearance seizures differ from commonplace nonattendance seizures in the following ways:

- They are less normal.

- They last more.

- Jerking and different developments are progressively articulated.

- People are increasingly mindful of their

environment.

A great many people with atypical nonappearance seizures have neurologic variations from the norm or formative postponements. Atypical nonattendance seizures as a rule proceed into adulthood.

Status epilepticus

Convulsive status epilepticus is the most genuine seizure issue and is viewed as a health-related crisis in light of the fact that the seizure doesn't stop. Electrical releases happen all through the cerebrum, causing a summed-up tonic-clonic seizure.

Convulsive status epilepticus is analyzed when either of the following happens:

- A seizure lasts over 5 minutes
- People don't totally recapture awareness between at least two seizures

Individuals have seizures with exceptional muscle withdrawals and frequently can't inhale enough. Body temperature increments. Without quick treatment, the heart and cerebrum can move toward becoming overburdened and for all time harmed, now and again bringing about death.

Summed-up convulsive status epilepticus has numerous causes, including harming the head and unexpectedly halting an anti-seizure tranquilize.

Non-convulsive status epilepticus, another kind of status epilepticus, doesn't cause spasms. The seizures happen for 10 minutes or more. During the seizure, mental procedures (counting mindfulness) and additionally conduct are influenced. Individuals may seem befuddled or scattered. They might not be able to talk and may carry on nonsensically. Having non-convulsive status epilepticus expands the danger of creating convulsive status epilepticus. This kind of seizure requires brief conclusion and treatment.

Indications After a Seizure

At the point when a seizure stops, individuals may have a cerebral pain, sore muscles, bizarre sensations, perplexity, and significant weariness. These eventual outcomes are known as the post-ictal state. In certain individuals, one side of the body is feeble after a seizure, and the shortcoming keeps going longer than the seizure (a confusion called Todd loss of motion).

A great many people don't recall what occurred during the seizure (a condition called post-ictal amnesia).

Difficulties

Seizures may have genuine outcomes. Serious, fast muscle compressions can cause wounds, including broken bones. Unexpected loss of cognizance can cause genuine damage because of falls and mishaps. Individuals may have various seizures without bringing about genuine mind harm. In any case, seizures that repeat and cause spasms may inevitably impede insight.

In the event that seizures are not well-controlled,

individuals might be not able get a driver's permit. They may experience issues keeping a vocation or getting protection. They might be socially vilified. Subsequently, their personal satisfaction might be generously decreased.

In the event that seizures are not totally controlled, individuals are a few times bound to pass on than the individuals who don't have seizures.

A couple of individuals kick the bucket all of a sudden for no clear reason—an entanglement called abrupt surprising passing in epilepsy. This issue happens around evening time or during rest. Hazard is most noteworthy for individuals who have visit seizures, particularly summed-up tonic-clonic seizures.

Analysis

- A specialist's assessment
- If the individual has never had a seizure, blood and different tests, imaging of the mind, and generally electroencephalography
- If a seizure issue has just been analyzed, typically blood tests to quantify levels of antiseizure drugs

Specialists analyze a seizure issue when individuals have at any rate two unjustifiable seizures that happen at various occasions. The finding depends on indications and the perceptions of observers. Manifestations that recommend a seizure incorporate loss of awareness, muscle fits that shake the body, loss of bladder control, abrupt disarray, and powerlessness to focus. In any case, seizures cause such indications substantially less regularly than the vast majority think. A short loss of cognizance is bound to swoon (syncope) than a seizure.

Individuals are typically assessed in a crisis division. On the off chance that a seizure issue has just been analyzed and individuals have totally recuperated, they might be assessed in a specialist's office.

History and Physical Assessment

An observer report of the scene can be useful to specialists. An onlooker can depict precisely what occurred, though individuals who have a scene typically can't. Specialists need to have a precise depiction, including the following:

- How quick the scene began
- Whether it included unusual muscle developments, (for example, fits of the head, neck, or facial muscles), tongue gnawing, slobbering, loss of bladder or gut control, or muscle hardening
- How long it kept going
- How rapidly the individual recuperated

A speedy recuperation recommends blacking out instead of a seizure. Disarray that goes on for a long time to hours after cognizance shows a seizure happened.

In spite of the fact that observers might be excessively terrified during the seizure to recall all subtleties, whatever they can recollect can help. In the event that happens, to what extent a seizure lasts ought to be planned with a watch or other gadget. Seizures that last just 1 or 2 minutes can appear to go on until the end of time.

Specialists additionally need to comprehend what individuals experienced before the scene: regardless of whether they had a hunch or cautioning that something strange was going to occur and in the case of anything, for example, certain sounds or glimmering lights, appeared to trigger the scene.

Specialists get some information about potential reasons for seizures, for example, the following:

- Whether individuals have had a confusion that can cause seizures or head damage

- Which drugs (counting liquor) they are taking or have as of late halted

- For individuals who are ingesting medications to control seizures, regardless of whether they are consuming the medications as prescribed

- Whether they are getting enough rest (not getting enough rest can make seizures bound to happen in certain individuals)

A careful physical assessment is finished. It might give hints to the reason for the side effects.

Testing

When a seizure is analyzed, more tests are normally

expected to recognize the reason. Individuals known to have a seizure issue may not need tests, aside from a blood test to quantify the degrees of the anti-seizure drugs they are taking.

In other individuals, blood tests are frequently done to gauge the degrees of substances, for example, sugar, calcium, sodium, and magnesium and to decide if the liver and kidneys are working regularly. An example of pee might be investigated to check for recreational medications that may not be accounted for. Such medications can trigger a seizure.

Electrocardiography might be done to check for a strange heart mood. Since an irregular heart musicality can enormously decrease blood stream (and hence oxygen supply) to the cerebrum, it can trigger loss of cognizance and once in a while a seizure or side effects that take after a seizure.

Imaging of the mind is normally done immediately to check for draining or a stroke. Ordinarily, figured tomography (CT) is done, yet attractive reverberation imaging (MRI) might be finished. The two tests can recognize mind variations from the norm that could be causing seizures. X-ray gives clearer, progressively nitty gritty pictures of the mind tissue; however, it isn't in every case promptly accessible.

In the event that specialists presume a mind disease, for example, meningitis or encephalitis, a spinal tap (lumbar cut) is normally done.

Electroencephalography (EEG) can help affirm the

analysis. EEG is an effortless, safe methodology that records electrical action in the cerebrum. Specialists look at the account (electroencephalogram) for proof of unusual electrical releases. Since the chronicle time is constrained, EEG can miss variations from the norm, and results might be typical, even in individuals who have a seizure issue. EEG is here and there planned after individuals have been denied of rest for 18 to 24 hours since absence of rest makes strange releases bound to happen.

EEG might be rehashed on the grounds that when done every second or even a third time, it might distinguish the reason, which was missed in the first run till the test was finished.

On the off chance that the determination is as yet unsure, particular tests, for example, video-EEG observing, should be possible at an epilepsy focus.

For video-EEG observing, individuals are admitted to an emergency clinic for 2 to 7 days, and EEG is done while they are video-taped. In the event that individuals are taking an anti-seizure medicate, it is frequently halted to improve the probability of a seizure. On the off chance that a seizure happens, specialists contrast the EEG recording and the video recording of the seizure. They may then have the option to distinguish the kind of seizure and the territory of the cerebrum where the seizure started.

Mobile EEG empowers specialists record mind movement for quite a long time at once—while individuals are at home. It might be valuable if seizures repeat in individuals who can't be admitted to the medical clinic for quite a while.

Guess

With treatment, 33% of individuals with epilepsy are free from seizures, and most become seizure-free soon after beginning treatment. In another third, seizures repeat not exactly half as regularly as they did before treatment. On the off chance that seizures are well-controlled with medications, around 60 to 70% of individuals can inevitably quit taking anti-seizure sedatives and remain sans seizure.

Epileptic seizures are viewed as settled when individuals have been sans seizure for a long time and have not taken anti-seizure drugs throughout the previous 5 years of that timespan.

Treatment

- Elimination of the reason if conceivable

- General measures

- Drugs to control seizures

- Sometimes medical procedure or different techniques if medications are incapable

On the off chance that the reason for the seizures can be distinguished and disposed of, no extra treatment is vital. For instance, if a low (glucose) level (hypoglycemia) caused the seizure, glucose is given, and the turmoil causing the low level is dealt with. Other treatable causes incorporate a disease, certain tumors, and an unusual sodium level.

In the event that the reason can't be wiped out, general measures in addition to medications are typically adequate to treat seizure issue. On the off chance that medications are incapable, medical procedure might be prescribed.

General Measures

Exercise is typically prescribed and social exercises are empowered. Be that as it may, individuals who have a seizure issue may need to make a few changes. For instance, they might be encouraged to do the following:

- Eliminate or reduce their intake of mixed refreshments
- •Avoid the use of recreational medications
- Refrain from exercises in which an unexpected loss of awareness could bring about genuine damage, for example, washing in a bath, climbing, swimming, or working force devices

After seizures are controlled (regularly for in any event a half year), they can do these exercises if satisfactory precautionary measures are taken. For instance, they should swim just when lifeguards are available.

In many states, laws disallow individuals with a seizure issue from driving until they have been free of seizures for at any rate a half year to 1 year.

A relative or dear companion and colleagues ought to be prepared to help if a seizure happens. Endeavoring to put an item, (for example, a spoon) in the individual's mouth to secure the individual's tongue ought not to be attempted. Such endeavors can accomplish more damage than anything else. The teeth might be harmed, or the individual may chomp the assistant accidentally as the jaw muscles contract. Be that as it may, partners ought to do the following during a seizure:

- Protect the individual from falling

- Loosen dress around the neck

- •Place a cushion under the head

- Roll the individual over to the other side

On the off chance that a pad is inaccessible, aides can put their foot or spot a thing of attire under the individual's head. Individuals who lose cognizance ought to be moved onto one side to straightforwardness breathing and help keep them from breathing in regurgitation or spit. Breathing in regurgitation or salivation can prompt desire pneumonia (a lung contamination brought about by breathing in spit, stomach substance, or both).

Individuals who have had a seizure ought not be disregarded until they have stirred totally, are never again confounded, and can move about regularly. For the most part, their PCP ought to be told.

Anti-Seizure Drugs

Anti-seizure drugs (additionally called anticonvulsants or antiepileptic drugs) lessen the danger of having another seizure. Typically, they are recommended just if individuals have had more than one seizure and if reversible causes, for example, low glucose, have been discounted or totally revised. Anti-seizure medications are normally not recommended when individuals have had just one summed-up seizure.

Most anti-seizure medications are taken by mouth.

Anti-seizure medications can totally stop seizures in around 33% of individuals who have them and enormously lessen the recurrence of seizures in another third. Very nearly 66% of individuals who react to anti-seizure medications can inevitably quit taking them without having a backslide. In any case, if anti-seizure medications are insufficient, individuals are alluded to a seizure focus and assessed for medical procedure.

There are a wide range of kinds of anti-seizure drugs. Which one is compelling relies upon the kind of seizure and different components. For the vast majority, taking one anti-seizure drug, typically the first or second one attempted, controls seizures. On the off chance that seizures repeat, distinctive anti-seizure medications are attempted. In such cases, figuring out which medication is compelling may take a while. A few people need to consume a few medications, which builds the danger of reactions. Some anti-seizure medications are not utilized alone, however just with other anti-seizure drugs.

Specialists take care to decide the proper portion for every individual. The best portion is the littlest portion that stops all seizures while having the least reactions. Specialists get some information about reactions, and at that point change the portion if necessary. Here and there specialists additionally measure the degree of anti-seizure medicate in the blood.

Anti-seizure medications ought to be accepted similarly as endorsed. Individuals who ingest medications to control seizures should see a specialist normally for portion change and ought to consistently wear a restorative ready wrist trinket engraved with the sort of seizure issue and the medication being taken.

Anti-seizure medications can meddle with the adequacy of different medications, and the other way around. Subsequently, individuals should ensure their PCP knows every one of the medications they are taking before they start taking anti-seizure drugs. They ought to likewise converse with their primary care physician and conceivably their drug specialist before they start consuming some other medications, including over-the-counter medications.

After seizures are controlled, individuals take the anti-seizure medicate until they have been sans seizure for in any event 2 years. At that point, the portion of the medication might be diminished continuously, and the medication in the long run halted. On the off chance that a seizure repeats after the anti-seizure medication is halted, individuals may need to take an anti-seizure sedative uncertainly. Seizures for the most part repeat inside 2 years in the event that they are going to.

Seizures are bound to repeat in individuals who have had any of the following:

- A seizure issue since adolescence
- The need to take more than one anti-seizure medication to be without seizure
- Seizures while taking an anti-seizure tranquilizer
- Focal seizures or myoclonic seizures
- Abnormal EEG results inside the earlier year
- Structural harm to the mind—for instance, by a stroke or tumor

Anti-seizure drugs, albeit successful, may have symptoms. Many reason laziness, however some may make kids hyperactive. For some anti-seizure drugs, blood tests are done intermittently to decide if the medication is debilitating kidney or liver capacity or lessening the quantity of platelets. Individuals taking anti-seizure medications ought to know about conceivable symptoms and ought to counsel their PCP whenever there's any hint of reactions.

For ladies who have a seizure issue and are pregnant, taking an anti-seizure medication expands the danger of prematurely delivering or of having a child with a birth deformity of the spinal line, spine, or cerebrum. Be that as it may, halting the anti-seizure medication might be progressively unsafe to the lady and the child. Having a summed-up seizure during pregnancy can harm or murder the hatchling. Therefore, proceeding to take an anti-seizure medication is typically prescribed. All ladies who are of childbearing age and taking an anti-seizure medication should take folate enhancements to lessen the danger of having an infant with a birth deformity.

Crisis Treatment

Crisis treatment to stop the seizures is required for:

- • Status epilepticus
- • Seizures that last over 5 minutes

Huge dosages of at least one anti-seizure drugs (regularly beginning with a benzodiazepine, for example, lorazepam) are given intravenously as fast as conceivable to stop the seizure. The sooner anti-seizure medications are begun, the better and the more effectively seizures are controlled.

Measures to avoid wounds are taken during the drawn-out seizure. Individuals are checked to ensure breathing is satisfactory. On the off chance that it isn't, a cylinder is embedded to help with breathing—a method called intubation.

On the off chance that seizures continue, a general soporific is given to stop them.

Medical Procedure

On the off chance that individuals keep on having seizures while taking at least two anti-seizure drugs or on the off chance that they can't endure symptoms of the medications, cerebrum medical procedure might be finished. These individuals are tried at specific epilepsy focuses to decide if medical procedure can help. Testing may incorporate MRI of the mind, video-EEG checking, and the following:

- Functional MRI: To figure out which territories in the cerebrum are causing seizures (called seizure foci)

- Single-photon discharge CT (SPECT): To check for zones with expanded blood stream around the hour of a seizure, which may show which regions in the mind are causing seizures

- EEG joined with magnets utilized for imaging (attractive source imaging): Also to help figure out which zones in the mind are causing seizures

In the event that an imperfection in the cerebrum, (for example, a scar) can be recognized as the reason and is kept to a little zone, precisely evacuating that zone can wipe out seizures in up to 60% of individuals, or medical procedure may lessen the seriousness and recurrence of seizures.

Precisely cutting the nerve strands that associate the different sides of the cerebrum (corpus callosum) may help individuals who have seizures that start in a few zones of the mind or that spread to all pieces of the mind rapidly. This methodology for the most part has no apparent symptoms. Be that as it may, regardless of whether medical procedure diminishes the recurrence and seriousness of seizures, numerous individuals need to keep on taking anti-seizure drugs. Notwithstanding, they can more often than not take lower dosages or less medications.

Incitement of the Vagus Nerve

Electrical incitement of the tenth cranial nerve (vagus nerve) can diminish the quantity of central beginning seizures by more than one half in about 40% of individuals who have central beginning seizures. This treatment is utilized when seizures proceed in spite of utilization of anti-seizure drugs and when medical procedure isn't a probability.

The vagus nerve is thought to have circuitous associations with territories of the mind regularly engaged with causing seizures. For this technique, a gadget that resembles a heart pacemaker (vagus nerve trigger) is embedded under the left collarbone and is associated with the vagus nerve in the neck with a wire that keeps running under the skin. The gadget causes a little lump under the skin. The activity is done on an outpatient premise and takes around 1 to 2 hours.

The gadget is customized to intermittently animate the vagus nerve. Additionally, individuals are given a magnet, which they can use to animate the vagus nerve when they sense that a seizure is going to start. Vagus nerve incitement is utilized notwithstanding anti-seizure drugs.

Reactions of vagal nerve incitement incorporate raspiness, hack, and extending of the voice when the nerve is animated.

Incitement of the Cerebrum

The responsive neurostimulation framework is a gadget that resembles a heart pacemaker. It is embedded inside the skull. The gadget is associated by wires to a couple of regions in the cerebrum that are causing the seizures. This framework screens the cerebrum's electrical movement. At the point when it distinguishes irregular electrical movement, it animates the zones of the cerebrum that are causing the seizures. The point is to re-establish ordinary electrical action in the mind before a seizure can happen.

The responsive neurostimulation framework is utilized notwithstanding anti-seizure drugs. It is utilized when grown-ups have central beginning seizures that are not constrained by medications. It can lessen the recurrence of seizures in these individuals.

Medical procedure to embed the framework requires general anesthesia and normally takes 2 to 4 hours. Numerous individuals can return home the following day, while some need to remain in the medical clinic for as long as 3 days. Numerous individuals can come back to their day-by-day exercises inside a couple of days and come back to work in two to about a month.

Certain psychological issue can cause indications that take after seizures, called psychogenic nonepileptic seizures or pseudoseizures.

At the end of the day, you may react to a circumstance as compromising when you are really protected. In these circumstances, you can figure out how to supersede pointless cautious horrible responses of battle, flight, stop, or blackout.

Mind-Body Therapies for Vagus Nerve Disorders

Drawing in your social sensory system oversees vagus nerve issue. Your social sensory system is reinforced by rehashed practice which myelinates the nerve pathways. Myelination is the greasy covering on nerves that is created through rehashed use and prompts expanded speed and control.

Mixed States and the Vagus Nerve

When you realize how to connect with your social sensory system you can apply these aptitudes during times when you fondle keyed with tension or contracted into sorrow. Commitment of your social sensory system while prepared by your thoughtful sensory system enables you to get to your inventiveness, become lively, and hit the dance floor with the accessible vitality.

Then again, captivating your social sensory system when you feel shut somewhere around awful recollections may enable you to abrogate baseless cautious immobilizing responses. Here, you can concentrate on associating with your heart in a position of stillness or interfacing with a friend or family member for more prominent closeness. Such a mix is additionally significant to encourage ease during labor, nursing, or holding. Porges (2017) recommends that this mix can help you to associate with a general unbounded feeling of unity.

Tone Your Vagus Nerve

Mind-body treatments direct the vagus nerve and increment your versatility through "safe preparation and safe immobilization". This includes at first building up your ability to feel quiet, quiet, and associated. When you have a strong establishment of having the option to get to your social sensory system, you can gradually fabricate your resilience for troubling physiological enactment. This is cultivated by mixing social commitment with both activation and immobilization until you can restore a feeling of wellbeing with those sensory system states. After some time, you increment your ability to move all through various sensory system states.

Mind-body treatments and substantial brain research welcome you to all the while take care of your body sensations, breath, passionate experience, and your considerations. Furthermore, you center around detecting your outer condition which will enable you to perceive that you are sheltered at this very moment. A few practices include careful utilization of development (for example yoga stances, kendo, strolling reflection) and others, careful utilization of stillness (situated contemplation, unwinding, yoga nidra).

In Practice

Connecting with the vagus nerve during development or stillness can take into consideration distinctive social sensory system mixing for changing wellbeing needs and vitality levels. Follow the following 4-Part practice intended to enable you to recoup from vagus nerve issue:

Section 1: Find a Safe Space

Start by finding a spot where you realize you are sheltered to investigate this mind-body practice. Locate an agreeable position either standing, situated, or setting down. Check out your space; recognize viewable prompts that disclose to you that you are sheltered, at this very moment. Rehash to yourself these words all through the training, "I am protected, I am associated, I am quiet."

Section 2: Increase Sensory Awareness

Take a few long, full breaths. Notice the impressions of the breath in your body and the unpretentious developments made by your breath. Presently, carry your attention to the sound of your breath. Extend your tangible attention to see some other sensations in your body. Rehash the expression, "I am sheltered, I am associated, I am quiet." If anytime in the training you experience nervousness or different trouble, come back to stage one by checking out your space to advise yourself that you are protected at this point.

Section 3: Explore Mindful Mobilization

Presently, start to investigate expanding the force of your breath while moving your body. Possibly, you stand up into a functioning yoga pose. Maybe you walk energetically set up or around the room. You can even put on your main tune and move! Increment your heart rate only enough to see that your breath animates to help your development. Rehash your expression, "I am sheltered, I am associated, I am quiet" as you move your body. By and by, on the off chance that you experience any nervousness or different pain, check out your space to advise yourself that you are protected at this point.

Section 4: Explore Mindful Immobilization

The last advance of this training welcomes you to come back to stillness either standing, situated, or setting down. Permit your heart rate to back off. Give up your weight down toward the earth. Take long, full breaths; breathe out longer than you breathe in to start an unwinding reaction. Be still and mellow any pointless holding in your muscles. Rehash your expression, "I am sheltered, I am associated, I am quiet" as you interface with stillness. By and by, on the off chance that you experience any nervousness or different trouble, check out your space to advise yourself that you are sheltered at this point.

Glossopharyngeal Neuralgia (Throat Torment)

Neuralgia is serious torment brought about by damage or harm to a nerve. Be aware that the glossopharyngeal nerve happens to be the ninth (IX) cranial nerve. And it emerges inside the skull from the brainstem. It supplies sensation to the back of the throat and tongue and parts of the ear.

At the point when the glossopharyngeal nerve ends up disturbed, an assault of extreme electric stun like torment is felt in the back of the throat, tongue, tonsil, or ear. Glossopharyngeal agony can be like trigeminal neuralgia – and misdiagnosed. Make certain to see a neurosurgeon who represents considerable authority in facial agony who can make the differentiation.

What Are the Side Effects?

Patients portray an assault as a copying or poking torment, or as an electrical stun that may last a couple of moments or minutes. Gulping, biting, talking, hacking, yawning, or snickering can trigger an assault. A few people portray the sentiment of a sharp item held up in the throat. The agony for the most part has the following highlights:

The torment, more often than not, has the following highlights:

1. 1Affects one side of the throat

2. 2an be present for a few days or weeks, trailed by a reduction for a considerable length of time or years

About 10% of patients likewise have possibly dangerous scenes of heart inconsistencies brought about by association of the close-by vagus nerve, for example,

- slow beat

- sudden drop in circulatory strain

- fainting (syncope)

- seizures

What Are the Causes?

Many accept that the defensive sheath of the nerve crumbles, sending anomalous messages. Like static in a phone line, these variations from the norm upset the ordinary sign of the nerve and cause torment. Regularly, the harm is from a vein packing the nerve. Different causes include maturing, various sclerosis, and close by tumors.

Who Is Influenced?

Glossopharyngeal neuralgia is uncommonly contrasted with other facial torment disorders. It happens marginally more in ladies than men; typically middle age and more established.

How Is a Finding Made?

At the point when an individual first encounters

throat torment, an essential consideration specialist or dental specialist is frequently advised. On the off chance that the torment requires further assessment, a nervous system specialist or a neurosurgeon might be suggested.

The conclusion of neuralgia is made after cautiously evaluating the patient's indications. In the event that glossopharyngeal neuralgia is suspected, the specialist will endeavor to trigger a scene by contacting the back of the throat with a swab. On the off chance that that causes torment, a topical analgesic is applied to the back of the throat and the specialist will attempt the agony boost once more. On the off chance that torment isn't activated while the region is numb, glossopharyngeal neuralgia is analyzed.

Different tests may incorporate a MRI or MRA to search for tumors or a vein compacting the nerve.

What Medicines Are Accessible?

An assortment of medicines are accessible, including drug, medical procedure, needle systems, and radiation. First-line treatment is normally prescription. At the point when prescriptions refuse to control torment or cause heinous symptoms, a neurosurgeon might be advised to talk about different strategies.

Drug

Over-the-counter medications, for example, headache medicine and ibuprofen are not compelling against neuralgia torment.

Anticonvulsants, for example, carbamazepine (Tegretol), gabapentin (Neurontin), are utilized to control torment. In the event that the medication starts to lose viability, the specialist may build the portion or change to another kind. Symptoms may include sluggishness, shakiness, sickness, skin rash, and blood issue. Along these lines, patients are observed with intermittent blood tests to guarantee that the medication levels stay safe. Numerous medication treatments might be important to control torment (e.g., Tegretol and amitriptyline).

A few people deal with the torment trigger by applying a fluid xylocaine to the tonsil territory and incidentally desensitizing it so they can eat and swallow.

Medical Procedure

Microvascular Decompression (MVD) is a medical procedure to tenderly reroute the vein from compacting the nerve by cushioning the supply route with a wipe. Medical procedure is performed under general anesthesia and requires a 1 to multi-day emergency clinic remain.

During medical procedure, a 1-inch opening, called a craniotomy, is made in the skull behind the ear. This uncovers the nerve at its association with the brainstem. A vein (at times a tumor) is frequently discovered compacting the nerve. After the nerve is liberated from pressure, it is ensured with a little Teflon wipe. The wipe stays in the cerebrum for all time.

MVD gives relief from discomfort in 85% of patients. The significant advantage of MVD is that it causes next to zero gulping or voice symptoms. In any case, there is a 5% danger of death because of control of the close-by vagus nerve, which can cause issues with pulse and circulatory strain.

MVD + Nerve Rhizotomy is a medical procedure to move the supply route (whenever found) and cut the nerve root at its association with the brainstem. Like the MVD medical procedure, a little opening is made in the back of the skull. On the off chance that a vein packing the nerve isn't found, or on the off chance that it can't be effectively moved, the specialist may pick to cut the nerve. The glossopharyngeal nerve is recognized and cut. At that point an incitement test is utilized to distinguish just the tactile foundations of the vagus nerve. The tactile root strands, which transmit the agony sign to the cerebrum, are cut off. The whole vagus nerve isn't cut.

MVD + rhizotomy gives 96% long haul relief from discomfort [1]. The potential reactions of rhizotomy are roughness of voice, trouble gulping (dysphagia), and loss of taste sensation.

Needle Techniques

Percutaneous Stereotactic Radiofrequency Rhizotomy (PSR) is an insignificantly obtrusive methodology that arrives at the nerve through the cheek without a skin cut or skull opening. The outpatient method is performed under nearby anesthesia and light sedation. Patients return home that day.

An empty needle is embedded through the skin of

the cheek into the glossopharyngeal nerve at the base of the skull. A cathode passes a warming current to obliterate a portion of the glossopharyngeal nerve filaments that produce torment. This method is ordinarily suggested for those with agony brought about by throat or neck disease.

Radiation

The objective of radiation treatment is to harm the nerve root to interfere with the agony signals from arriving at the mind. Stereotactic radiosurgery is a non-invasive outpatient technique that utilizations high-vitality pillars to decimate a portion of the glossopharyngeal nerve filaments. A stereotactic cover or edge is connected to the patient's head to decisively find the nerve on a MRI filter and to hold the head flawlessly as yet during treatment. Profoundly engaged light emissions are conveyed to the nerve root. In the weeks after treatment, sore (damage) steadily occurs where the radiation happened.

Help with discomfort may not happen quickly, but instead bit by bit after some time. Patients stay taking drugs for a while following treatment to control the agony while the radiation produces results.

Clinical Preliminaries

Clinical preliminaries are research examinations in which new medicines—drugs, diagnostics, methodology, and different treatments—are tried in individuals to check whether they are sheltered and compelling. Research is continually being led to improve the standard of restorative consideration.

CHAPTER FIVE

HOW TO KNOW IF YOUR VAGUS NERVE IS INJURED OR COMPRESSED

Your fringe nerves are the connections between your cerebrum and spinal rope and the remainder of your body. Fringe nerves are delicate and effectively harmed. Nerve damage can influence your cerebrum's capacity to speak with your muscles and organs. Harm to the fringe nerves is called fringe neuropathy.

Extending or pushing on a nerve can cause damage. The nerves additionally might be harmed because of other wellbeing conditions that influence the nerves, for example, diabetes or Guillain-Barre disorder.

In carpal passage disorder, weight on the middle nerve in the wrist causes harm. Or on the other hand the nerves might be squashed, cut, or harmed in a mishap, for example, games damage or an auto collision.

Now and then in a fringe nerve damage, either the strands or the protection are harmed. These wounds are bound to recuperate. In increasingly extreme fringe nerve wounds both the filaments and the protection are harmed, and the nerve might be totally cut. These kinds of wounds are exceptionally hard to treat and recuperation may not be conceivable. For instance, in the event that you feel shivering or deadness or create shortcoming in your leg, arm, shoulder or hand, you may have harmed at least one nerves in a mishap. You may likewise encounter comparative side effects if a nerve is being packed because of elements, for example, a limited path, tumor or different sicknesses.

It's critical to get restorative consideration for a fringe nerve damage as quickly as time permits since nerve tissue now and then can be fixed. Early analysis and treatment now and again can avert difficulties and lasting damage.

Signs Your Vagal Nerve Is Powerless

Vagal nerve sign can wind up feeble or the nerve can move toward becoming bothered because of overwhelming metal poisonous quality, poor stance, Hiatal hernias, abundance liquor, stress, and mind injury (a solitary blackout can cause powerless vagal nerve tone). Indications of powerless vagal nerve tone or misregulated terminating of the vagal nerve can cause the following manifestations:

- Lack of a muffle reflex
- Slow absorption: nourishment sits in your stomach excessively long. This can cause heartburn or GERD, swelling, or clogging.
- Inability to unwind
- Heart palpitations
- Insomnia

Probably the best indication of solid vagal tone is the point at which your pulse increases somewhat with inward breath, and moderate marginally with exhalation.

How Would You Reinforce the Vagal Nerve?

About 60% of vagal nerve tone is dictated by hereditary qualities; however, there is a strong 40% that we can affect! Become familiar with various approaches to fortify and animate the vagus nerve.

Fun truth: You CAN overstimulate the vagus nerve, and this is the most widely recognized reason for blacking out. On the off chance that you've at any point blacked out or felt tipsy in the wake of giving blood or getting a shot, you likely experienced "vasovagal syncope." At the point when you are under exceptionally high pressure your vagus nerve turns out to be excessively invigorated and your pulse drops rapidly making you feel woozy or lose cognizance. It's just brief, and sitting or resting for the most part settles the inclination rapidly.

Frail vagal nerve tone is connected to aggravation,

wretchedness, forlornness and cardiovascular failures. We need to ensure our vagal nerves are solid! The following all invigorate the vagus nerve only enough to be exceptionally restorative, however less to cause blacking out but rather more these are not profoundly distressing occasions.

1.   Gargling

Gargling animates the vagus nerve, albeit dainty swishing won't do it. You have to wash noisily and forcefully, to the point of nearly choking. Doing this day by day will help increment the responsiveness of your vagal nerve to direct unwinding, absorption, digestion, and that's just the beginning.

2.   Playing Instruments

Fascinating   research   with   didgeridoos demonstrated that playing the instrument is compelling in treating obstructive rest issue and rest apnea through its solid incitement of the vagus nerve. Further research demonstrates that various provocative conditions were additionally improved. Most wind instruments animate the vagus nerve.

3.   Yogic or Deep Breathing

Holding your breath for 6-8 checks animates the vagus nerve. Attempt this: Use your stomach to take in for a check of 6, hold for 6-8, and breathe out gradually through pressed together lips for 6-8 tallies to get your vagus terminating. It's essential to have the option to feel your stomach (that line between your stomach and ribs) going all over with every breath. It takes around 10 minutes of this breathing to feel the profoundly loosening-up impacts of the vagal nerve incitement.

4.   Meditation

Learning cherishing graciousness reflections improves vagal tone. This is because of its impact on positive feelings and positive associations. The more positive feelings and associations we have, the more grounded our vagal tone. Download my free reflection present.

5.   Acupuncture

Acupuncture is astonishing for managing vagal nerve reaction. Electroacupuncture utilizes a little machine that emanates an effortless electromagnetic heartbeat. The electromagnetic heartbeat feels like a slight humming or tapping and isn't horrendous. Following 20-30 minutes of this, you will leave the workplace feeling unbelievably loose. That vagal nerve incitement will help direct every one of the procedures constrained by the vagal nerve, which at this point you know is a whoop dee doo!

Bioelectronics is a developing field of medication where little gadgets are embedded to animate diverse sensory system pathways. This effectively treats a scope of maladies and provocative side effects. This is energizing and approving of needle therapy which uses needles and other things to invigorate the sensory system at various focuses to treat a scope of illness and incendiary side effects. On the off chance that you need to be on the bleeding edge of logical research, and stay away from medical procedure to embed a metal gadget, attempt the less intrusive way, needle therapy.

CHAPTER SIX

HEALTH BENEFITS OF THE NERVE'S

STIMULATION

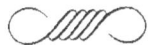

Aggravation is the fundamental reason for most infections as the insusceptible framework dispatches a fiery reaction to secure cells when it detects peril. In any case, identifying the underlying reason for that irritation can prove to be the more noteworthy test.

The vagus nerve associates with many body frameworks and impacts fundamental irritation and generally speaking wellbeing.

Investigating the Vagus Nerve and Its Functions

This article looks at why the vagus nerve is basic and its capacities to add to wellbeing, including:

- Why the vagus nerve is significant
- How the vagus nerve impacts wellbeing

- Signs and indications of vagus nerve brokenness
- agus nerve stimulation and its advantages
- A significant note on gluten and the vagus nerve

Why the Vagus Nerve Is Important

The vagus nerve reaches out from its underlying foundations in the cerebellum and brainstem, twists through the body, and branches on various occasions to innervate the majority of the following significant organs:

- the pharynx
- larynx
- heart
- esophagus
- stomach
- small digestive tract and
- large digestive tract up to its splenic flexure

This all-encompassing arrive at results in the vagus nerve assuming a job in capacities, for example, taste, gulping, discourse, pulse, processing, and discharge.

The vagus nerve fills in as a vital individual from the parasympathetic sensory system, or PNS, which related with physiological exercises ordered as, "rest and summary."

As its name infers, the PNS works in quieting the body down and processing nourishment to re-establish the body's vitality supply among different capacities. To accomplish this, the vagus nerve speaks with its related organs by discharging a synapse called acetylcholine which encourages pulse guideline, blood glucose balance, pulse, taste, processing, breathing, crying, perspiring, kidney work, bile discharge, salivation emission, female ripeness, and climaxes.

Hormones all through the body are likewise drawn in with the vagus nerve. Insulin diminishes glucose discharge from the liver to invigorate the vagus nerve though thyroid hormone, T3, animates the vagus nerve to expand hunger and the creation of ghrelin. Ghrelin additionally animates the vagus nerve to expand hunger.

Vagus nerve capacity is basic to the arrival of oxytocin, testosterone, and vasoactive intestinal peptide. The generation of development hormone discharging hormone, GHRH, and the initiation of parathyroid hormone for changing over nutrient D3 to dynamic nutrient D additionally depend on the vagus nerve.

Mental and Physical Health: How the Vagus Nerve Impacts

In spite of the fact that the vagus nerve influences organs outside of the focal sensory system, or CNS, which comprises of the mind and spinal rope, recall that the vagus nerve is established in the brainstem and cerebellum. Ideal vagus nerve capacity, or "high vagal tone list," is related with solid social associations, positive feelings, and better physical wellbeing. People with low vagal tone list experience melancholy, coronary episodes, depression, adverse emotions, and stroke.

Mind wellbeing and gut wellbeing impact each other and the vagus nerve is accurately the connection between the two. The vagal tone list can be thought of as the body's "hunch" that gets passed on straightforwardly to the mind and creates a criticism circle of greater energy or greater cynicism.

Developing investigations demonstrate that the vagal tone record is dictated by sign discharged from the invulnerable framework called cytokines. Research is in progress to all the more likely see how animating the vagus nerve offers the potential for treating incendiary conditions, for example, rheumatoid joint inflammation, without the utilization of pharmaceutical medications.

Signs and Symptoms of Vagus Nerve Dysfunction

Given the broad associations between the cerebrum and gut by means of the vagus nerve and its branches, there are various areas helpless against brokenness. These locales can be assembled into three primary regions:

- Communication inside the cerebrum

- Communication from the cerebrum to different organs

- Communication from different organs to the cerebrum

Contingent upon which territory is harassed, vagus

nerve brokenness may show as:

- Aggression
- Anxiety
- Brain haze
- Chronic irritation
- Delayed stomach exhausting
- Depression
- Difficulty gulping
- Dizziness or blacking out
- Fatigue
- Heart rate changes (high or low)
- Heartburn
- Irritable Bowel Syndrome (IBS)
- Vitamin B12 inadequacy
- Weight gain

Left undiscovered or untreated, vagus nerve brokenness can prompt progressively genuine sicknesses including:

- Alcohol habit
- Autism
- Bulimia
- Cancer
- Chronic cardiovascular breakdown
- Fibromyalgia

- Heart sickness
- Leaky Gut Syndrome
- Memory issue or Alzheimer's sickness
- Migraines
- Mood issue
- Multiple Sclerosis (MS)
- Obesity
- Obsessive Compulsive Disorder (OCD)
- Poor blood course
- Tinnitus

Staying away from maladies and way of life decisions that harm the vagus nerve is fundamental to keeping the above signs and side effects under control. These include liquor addiction, nervousness, diabetes, exhaustion, physical harm to the vagus nerve, poor stance, and stress.

Vagus Nerve Stimulation and Its Benefits

Vagus nerve brokenness normally results from a low vagal tone file, so animating the vagus nerve can work as a treatment for the signs, manifestations, and illnesses recorded previously. Huge numbers of these types of treatment speak to way of life changes meaning it is protected to embrace more than one of the following practices to expand the vagal tone record.

- Add fish to the eating routine

The EPA and DHA found in fish invigorate the

vagus nerve to build pulse changeability and lower pulse. These impacts can be gotten from a fish oil supplement also.

- Become a yogi

Yoga supports state of mind and brings down tension as well as builds vagus nerve and parasympathetic framework movement. The moderate, profound breathing related with yoga actuates exceptionally touchy weight receptors in the heart and neck called baroreceptors which send sign to the cerebrum telling it to initiate the vagus nerve.

- Build social associations

Research demonstrates social connections make people feel nearer to other people, and that feeling invigorates the vagus nerve.

- Chew gum

Biting gum supports the arrival of the hormone, CCK, from the gut which encourages correspondence from the vagus nerve to the cerebrum.

- Eat more fiber

Fiber expands GLP-1, a hormone that supports correspondence between the vagus nerve and cerebrum, eases back stomach purging and makes the body feel full more.

- Engage the larynx

Exercises like singing, washing, or in any event, initiating the muffle reflex, connect with the larynx along these lines animating the vagus nerve. For help with initiating the muffle reflex, utilize a tongue depressor or spoon.

- Exercise normally

Exercise animates the vagus nerve to invigorate gut stream subsequently profiting the vagal list alongside discharge.

- Fast irregularly

Irregular fasting lessens the quantity of calories expended. That decrease in calories causes pulse inconstancy to spike and digestion to plunge—two occasions that trigger vagus nerve work.

Discover an Acupuncturist

Conventional needle therapy, particularly to the ear, animates the vagus nerve.

- Get direct daylight

UVA beams increase the body's degrees of melanocyte animating hormone (MSH), another hormone that invigorates the vagus nerve. UVB beams increase the quantity of MSH receptors all through the body making it workable for much more MSH to tie.

- Incorporate petition each day

Studies show asking animates the vagus nerve by expanding diastolic circulatory strain and pulse inconstancy. These impacts improve by and large cardiovascular wellbeing.

- Laugh regularly

The association among chuckling and vagal tone was first found because of individuals blacking out from occasions that include the body hunkering down, for example, hacking, giggling, moving the guts, gulping, and peeing. The blacking out results from different disorders, including the vagus nerve, yet in solid people, chuckling supports better comprehension while counteracting coronary illness.

- Learn to cherish cold temperatures

Acclimating to temperatures colder than normal body temperature triggers the PNS vigorously by means of vagus nerve stimulation. This impact is best accomplished by drinking cold water, plunging the face in virus water, or washing up.

- Meditate day by day

Thinking to advance love and consideration inside the soul builds the vagal tone file. Om reciting is an elective technique for reflection that creates a similar impact.

- Practice Tai Chi

Studies show Tai Chi expands pulse fluctuation demonstrating it accomplishes this by actuating the vagus nerve.

- Have rubs regularly

Neck and foot back rubs animate the vagus nerve while decreasing the danger of seizures and coronary illness, separately. Entire body weight back rubs invigorate gut work which in a roundabout way enacts the vagus nerve.

- Sleep on the correct side

Lying on the back reduces vagus nerve actuation, yet dozing on the correct side shows more prominent vagus nerve incitement contrasted with left side dozing.

- Spend some time with Nervana

Nervana is a type of innovation intended to invigorate the vagus nerve by means of electrical waves matched up with music. Accessible as an uneven generator or double sided earphones, Nervana triggers synapse discharge from the cerebrum and prompts quiet inside the psyche and body.

- Supplement zinc and serotonin (5-HTP)

Zinc is essential to vagus nerve capacity, and numerous individuals are unconsciously inadequate in this mineral. Serotonin enacts the vagus nerve through a few distinct receptors in the body.

- Taking a probiotic: Optimising gut wellbeing is perfect for expanding vagus nerve stimulation. Taking a probiotic can guarantee this particularly the probiotic, Lactobacillus rhamnosus, which improves the capacity of GABA receptors for the vagus nerve in creature contemplates.

- Try a bowel purge

Assisting the development of the guts grows the digestion tracts and enacts vagus nerve movement.

- Use Pulsed Electromagnetic Field (PEMF) treatment

Research affirms that attractive fields animate the vagus nerve by expanding pulse fluctuation. Utilizing a gadget that invigorates beat attractive field waves straightforwardly on the gut, head, and neck will focus on the vagus nerve.

- Work the vocal harmonies

Reciting, murmuring, singing, talking, and other vocal harmony activities increase pulse changeability which enacts the vagus nerve.

Vagus Nerve and the Gluten: An Important Detail to Take Note Of

People delicate to gluten can encounter aggravation and mind issue including nervousness, mental imbalance, ADHD, bipolar issue, sadness, schizophrenia, Alzheimer's malady, or Parkinson's illness.

Such gluten affectability likewise disturbs gut wellbeing bringing about a diminished vagal file. In this way, stopping utilization of gluten is one more approach to invigorate the vagus nerve while supporting gut wellbeing and diminishing aggravation in the cerebrum.

Studies show vagus nerve incitement additionally brings down circulatory strain, diminishes pulse, lessens the body's reaction to stretch, and improves assimilation.

Be that as it may, it's as yet misty how comparative non-intrusive VNS is to an embedded VNS gadget, which is the reason Leonard's group is right now attempting to think about the two. "We record neural movement straightforwardly from the human cerebrum in patients with epilepsy, some of whom additionally as of now have embedded cervical VNS gadgets, and who volunteer to wear our ear gadget for a couple of minutes," said Leonard. This enables these specialists to check whether the incitement in the mind is comparative between these intrusive and non-obtrusive methodologies.

Vagus Nerve's Effect on Heftiness

The vagus nerve assumes a significant job in helping us feel satisfied after a dinner, which leads us to its connection to stoutness.

Basically, it's liable for sending that sign to quit eating when we're full to the cerebrum, making it mindful that we have momentary vitality to go through. This investigation demonstrates that the respectability of our vagal framework could in this way be connected to heftiness.

In the event that the vagus nerve isn't working ideally, our craving sign may not work as well as could be expected, causing indulging and weight gain.

It Keeps You Quiet

Like the arrival of the pressure hormone cortisol sends our bodies into "battle or flight" mode, the autonomic sensory system is liable for the "rest-and-summary" mode.

The vagus nerve sends sign to discharge prolactin, vasopressin, and oxytocin – all of which quiet us down. After some time, solid vagal tone can build pressure resistance which will prompt quicker recuperation time from disease, damage, stress, and passionate injury.

As indicated by research, vagus nerve incitement has promising outcomes for subduing nervousness and dread – in any event, when dread is unreasonably solid for presentation treatment. Vagus nerve incitement is a medicinal technique, during which electrical stuns are sent to the nerve, conveyed through an implantation. It's regularly used to treat epilepsy and sadness that is lethargic to average treatment, yet the extent of treatment is enlarging with new research that shows it could be useful to the individuals who experience the ill effects of incessant irritation.

The explanation this works is on the grounds that the electrical sign arrive at the cerebrum stem where they have an ideal beginning stage to send signs to different parts of the mind. The reason behind its solid connect to aggravation is connected to vagal tone. Like the heart, the "tone" or generally speaking soundness of it makes a difference, and it impacts numerous other real capacities.

In one investigation, an upward-winding dynamic was shown, connecting positive feeling, social association, and physical wellbeing – showed by vagal tone. Individuals who need to jump aboard with this hypothesis can build constructive feeling with adoring generosity contemplation which helps individuals self-produce an uplifting disposition toward oneself as well as other people.

Vagus nerve incitement (VNS) is a system used to treat epilepsy. It includes embedding a pacemaker-like gadget that produces beats of power to animate the vagus nerve. The vagus nerve is one of the 12 cranial nerves, the matched nerves that connect to the under surface of the cerebrum and hand-off data to and from the mind. Cranial nerve strands lead driving forces between the mind and different pieces of the cerebrum and different body structures, for the most part in the head and neck. The vagus nerve - the longest of the cranial nerves - likewise stretches out to organs in the chest and midriff.

What Are the Reactions of VNS?

The most widely recognized reactions of VNS include:

- Hoarseness
- Coughing
- Tingling in the neck and
- Problems gulping

For the most part, these happen just when the nerve is being animated, and are commonly mellow and will in general leave after some time.

When Is VNS Used to Treat Epilepsy?

- Brain cells impart by sending electrical flag in a

precise example. In individuals with epilepsy, this example is once in a while disturbed due either to damage or the individual's hereditary make-up, causing synapses to transmit flag in an uncontrolled manner. This makes over-fervor, to some degree like an electrical over-burden in the mind, prompting seizures. Seizures can be created by electrical motivations from all through the mind, called summed-up seizures, or from a little zone of the cerebrum, called fractional seizures.

- Most individuals with epilepsy can control their seizures with prescriptions called anticonvulsants or anti-seizure drugs.

- About 20% of individuals with epilepsy don't react to anti-seizure drugs.

- In a few cases, medical procedure to evacuate the piece of the mind causing the seizures might be utilized.

- VNS might be a treatment alternative for individuals whose seizures are not constrained by anti-seizure meds and who are not viewed as great contender for medical procedure; for instance, if their seizures are delivered all through the cerebrum (summed up).

Since it is so long and meandering (vagus actually means meandering in Latin), it controls and influences numerous pieces of our cognizant and oblivious substantial capacities, for example, keeping up a steady pulse, processing nourishment, and breathing. In this manner, brokenness of the nerve can prompt emotional episodes, and different ills, for example, seizures, b12 lacks, and corpulence.

Fortifying the capacity of the vagus nerve, then again, can improve conditions, for example, uneasiness, headaches, liquor compulsion, broken gut, Alzheimer's, malignant growth, coronary illness, and that's only the tip of the iceberg.

The following are a few methods that animate the solid capacity of the vagus nerve:

1. Rinsing

Rinsing animates similar muscles that the vagus nerve connects with. This can likewise improve memory work.

2. Developing Positive Relationships

Research demonstrates that just by thinking about our friends and family we can tone and reinforce the vagus nerve, along these lines receiving the numerous rewards that the nerve gives.

3. Introduction to the Cold

By drinking cold water or washing up, we reinforce our body's quieting framework (the parasympathetic framework) which occurs through the vagus nerve

4. Singing and Chanting

Singing as loud as possible builds pulse changeability and works the muscles in the back of your throat that associate with the vagus nerve.

5. Back Rubs

Aside from inclination astounding, a great back rub of the feet and neck activates the vagus nerve and can decrease seizures.

6. Satisfaction and Laughter

Having a decent snicker lifts your temperament, helps the resistant framework and animates the vagus nerve.

7. Yoga and Tai Chi

Both Yoga and Tai Chi give a large group of medical advantages and are especially useful for those battling with discouragement and uneasiness

8. Profound Breathing

Profound breathing animates the vagus nerve to lower pulse and pulse.

9. Exercise

Physical exercise is amazing both for gut stream and emotional wellness benefits, which both happen through the vagus nerve.

10. Unwinding

Practically, any loosening-up movement fortifies the vagus nerve's capacity to give healing to the body.

CHAPTER SEVEN

ANXIETY AND VAGUS NERVE

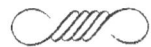

N ervousness can be a genuine doozy; it's outlandishly muddled, profoundly close to home, and ridiculously difficult to foresee. There are times when we think our uneasiness is behind us—that we are at long last one stage ahead—yet then something happens and we are on our heels once more, battling to return to a position of harmony and quiet. We are on the whole understudies of our uneasiness and that is the reason seeing precisely how our sensory system functions—and what we can do to quiet it—can be staggeringly enabling.

In any case, what does quieting your sensory system truly mean? Numerous individuals would depict it as easing back the pulse, developing the breath, and loosening up various muscles—however what really associates these sensations to the mind? You need to know more about the vagus nerve, the piece of the body that appears to clarify how our psyches control our bodies, how our bodies impact our brains and may give us the instruments we have to quiet them both.

Posttraumatic stress issue (PTSD) are encountered by numerous individuals. Ongoing catastrophic events, mass shootings, psychological oppressor assaults, and urban communities under attack add to the worldwide weight of PTSD which, as indicated by a recent report, influences 4–6% of the worldwide populace, despite the fact that most of injuries are identified with mishaps and sexual or physical savagery. Shockingly, there is no known fix, and flow medicines are not powerful for all patients.

A PTSD psychopharmacology working group as of late distributed their accord proclamation calling for quick activity to address the emergency in PTSD treatment, referring to three significant concerns. To start with, just two medications (sertraline and paroxetine) are endorsed by the US FDA for the treatment of PTSD. These meds decrease side effect seriousness, however may not create total reduction of side effects. The subsequent concern is identified with polypharmacy. PTSD patients are recommended prescriptions to address every one of their numerous extraordinary and assorted side effects including nervousness, trouble dozing, sexual brokenness, wretchedness and interminable torment, with lacking exact examinations of medication communications. The high comorbidity among PTSD and fixation gives further difficulties to pharmacotherapies. The third significant concern is the absence of headways in the treatment of PTSD; no new prescriptions have been endorsed since 2001.

Going past side effect alleviation, the 'best quality level' injury centered way to deal with treating PTSD pathology is introduction based treatment, where patients are presented to the tokens of the injury until they figure out how to connect these prompts with wellbeing. In spite of the fact that there is great proof for adequacy with this methodology, not all patients completely react to the treatment. Introduction treatment relies upon stifling the adapted dread memory, which is overwhelmed by another memory that is created through rehashed exposures. The patients with nervousness issue and PTSD show weaknesses in their capacity to quench adapted feelings of dread, which may meddle with advancement in treatment. Since the memory of the injury isn't lost at the same time, rather upgrades through treatments that rely upon new learned affiliations that rival horrible affiliations, the parity of the two recollections can move after some time, prompting backslide. Different difficulties incorporate the trouble in perceiving and smothering apprehension of every single molded boost, and a high dropout rate, which isn't astonishing given that shirking is one of the indications of PTSD.

Numerous creature investigate labs have tried endeavors to create adjunctive medications to quicken or improve the impacts of presentation based treatments. Spearheading work did by Michael Davis demonstrated that organization of the psychological improving medication d-cycloserine before presenting rodents to unreinforced molded signals upgraded annihilation, and he and his associates therefore deciphered the disclosure when they found that d-cycloserine likewise improved the impacts of presentation treatment in patients with explicit fears.

In any case, aftereffects of studies evaluating the impacts of psychological enhancers as subordinates to presentation treatment are blended on account of PTSD. A conceivable clarification is that medications given before introduction treatment sessions risk fortifying negative affiliations if presentation produces nervousness. Anxiolytic medications have been attempted, in light of proof that these medications ought to improve decency and decrease the tension reaction during introduction. Nonetheless, results show that anxiolytic medications don't improve the impacts of presentation treatment. One clarification is that the uneasiness reaction is required for accomplishment in introduction treatment since patients must learn not to fear their own dread reaction. Then again, similarly, as stress can improve the capacity of horrendous mishaps, the tension reaction may upgrade the combination of the termination memory. Predictable with this, anxiolytic medications will in general hinder memory combination. A perfect extra would take advantage of the systems that improve the union of horrendous recollections so as to advance elimination recollections that are similarly as solid, at the same time bypassing or maintaining a strategic distance from the aversive pressure reaction.

Developing proof proposes that vagus nerve

incitement (VNS) might be a gainful extra to introduction based treatments through its blending explicit improvement of memory combination and neural versatility. Enthusiasm for the vagus nerve (the tenth cranial nerve) as a neuromodulator originates from a very long while of research demonstrating that the vagus nerve fills in as an extension between the fringe autonomic sensory system and the cerebrum. It flags the mind during times of elevated thoughtful movement, advancing quick stockpiling of recollections that are significant for endurance. As a major aspect of the parasympathetic sensory system, initiation of the vagus nerve neutralizes the thoughtful pressure reaction.

VNS upgrades memory in rodents and people, proposing that blending VNS with unreinforced introduction to adapted signals may improve the union of the elimination memory. Predictable with this theory, we found that VNS upgraded elimination of molded dread in rodents. Broad proof shows that VNS advances neural versatility, particularly when it is combined with preparing, and this impact includes VNS regulation of the locus coeruleus noradrenergic framework. We have watched pliancy impacts in the termination related infralimbic prefrontal cortex – basolateral amygdala pathway in the wake of blending VNS with presentation to unreinforced molded prompts, proposing that VNS-improved elimination might be hearty, enduring, and less vulnerable to backslide.

In an ongoing report, we found that VNS likewise improved termination of molded dread in a rodent model of PTSD. These rodents express a considerable lot of the biomarkers and conduct phenotypes that are related with PTSD and, significantly, they are impervious to elimination of molded dread. We found that VNS organization during elimination sessions switched this termination disability and counteracted the arrival of dread. VNS-treated rodents likewise performed better on trial of tension, excitement, evasion, and social associations after some weeks, demonstrating that inversion of the elimination hindrance meant enhancements in other PTSD indications.

Moreover, interminable, unpaired VNS, as is utilized in the treatment of epilepsy and despondency, improved execution on the Hamilton Anxiety Scale in certain patients with tension issue, and diminished uneasiness like conduct in rodents. The impacts of VNS on termination in our examinations are not seen when the VNS is managed 30 min to 1 h in the wake of preparing. In this way, VNS alone isn't adequate to decrease the dread reaction.

These discoveries recommend that VNS may diminish nervousness; however, matching explicit pliancy and memory tweak is vital for elimination upgrade. Our ongoing, unpublished discoveries show that rodents are bound to investigate the open arms of a raised in addition to labyrinth following getting VNS, proposing that VNS produces an intense anxiolytic impact. Moreover, corticosterone levels expanded essentially in trick treated rodents following testing on the raised in addition to labyrinth, however such an expansion was not seen in VNS-treated rodents. This work ought to be imitated in different settings, yet it is an empowering initial move toward distinguishing an assistant treatment that may improve decency and adequacy in presentation based treatments.

The US FDA endorsed VNS as a strategy to forestall seizures in treatment-safe epilepsy patients in 1997, and in 2000 for treatment-safe discouragement. The vagus nerve innervates the core of the single tract, which is associated to the locus coeruleus and other limbic and forebrain cortical territories. VNS builds levels of monoamines in the cerebrum and the locus coeruleus assumes a job in VNS-initiated decrease of seizures. The current clinical routine with regards to VNS includes careful implantation of a terminal that is appended to one side cervical vagus nerve through an entry point in the neck. The cathode is associated by a lead that is burrowed under the skin to a heartbeat generator that is subcutaneously embedded in the chest. Careful inconveniences, for example, disease or vocal line impacts, happen in about 1% of patients. Less obtrusive ways to deal with animating the vagus nerve might be viable.

In the nineteenth century, the nervous system specialist James Leonard Corning created gadgets to invigorate the vagus nerve transcutaneously, while compacting the carotid supply route, and he watched a lessening in the recurrence and span of seizures. These were not controlled examinations and Corning deserted the methodology in view of reactions, for example, unsteadiness and syncope; be that as it may, transcutaneous VNS (t-VNS) has as of late recovered status as a clinical device. Noninvasive electrical incitement of the vagus can be controlled transcutaneously through the afferent auricular part of the nerve with cathodes cut to the concha district of the ear. With this t-VNS the electrical boost, with a force that is above tangible location yet underneath the agony limit, is applied through the skin to the open field of the auricular branch. Blended outcomes were found in an ongoing report inspecting t-VNS consequences for eradication of molded dread in people and clinical research on the utilization of t-VNS is constrained, however it is by all accounts sheltered and very much endured. Transcutaneous variants of VNS may give the advantages of VNS without the dangers of medical procedure; be that as it may, t-VNS isn't yet a setup treatment and assurance of its viability requires further examination.

VNS holds guarantee as an aide to introduction based treatments since it improves memory combination and advances synaptic pliancy while hosing the thoughtful pressure reaction. In spite of the fact that VNS has been utilized in people for more than two decades, the act of blending it with introduction treatment has not been tried in patients and numerous inquiries stay unanswered. 80% of the cervical filaments of the left vagus nerve are afferent tangible strands and preclinical examinations are right now in progress to inspect the general commitments of PNS versus CNS impacts of VNS. Singular contrasts in the nerve and in excitement state may cause inconstancy in impacts in human patients. Recognizable proof of a solid biomarker for VNS impacts would be useful for redoing parameters in treatment crosswise over people, and it might be utilized to check the potential adequacy of less obtrusive strategies for invigorating the vagus nerve, for example, t-VNS.

At last, it stays to be resolved whether VNS has an intense anxiolytic impact. As per our model, incitement of the vagus nerve sidesteps the thoughtful reaction to danger, while as yet advancing pliancy and quick union of enduring recollections. The job of the vagus nerve in the parasympathetic sensory system is to slow the thoughtful pressure reaction. Some proof shows that constant VNS decreases nervousness in people and in rodents. On the off chance that VNS can quickly decrease uneasiness, this may, or may not be helpful for presentation based treatments. It might meddle with the chance to quench the dread of the dread reaction. Then again, it might rush advancement and improve consistence by cutting off the relationship between introduction to injury prompts and the molded dread reaction during treatment. Studies are presently in progress to decide if diverse incitement parameters can be utilized to separate memory impacts of VNS from anxiolytic impacts.

During basic periods being developed, the cerebrum is more plastic than it is sometime down the road. Be that as it may, when under strain, the grown-up cerebrum can adjust. Quickly put away, durable recollections of sincerely stimulating occasions are a case of strong neural pliancy that can be cultivated in the grown-up cerebrum.

In 1890, William James expressed, "An encounter might be so energizing genuinely as nearly to leave a scar on the cerebral tissues". The neural pliancy that underlies horrible recollections can be versatile, decreasing the probability that a perilous conduct will be rehashed. Once in a while, awful recollections have maladaptive results, prompting tension or stress-related issue. We plan to bridle the capability of the vagus nerve to drive neural versatility during presentation treatment, while simultaneously intruding on the thoughtful battle-or-flight reaction. On the off chance that's fruitful, we will exploit instruments that exist to leave an enduring impact on the mind so as to mend the cerebral scars left by injury.

How is the Vagus Nerve Affecting Your Wellbeing?

In 1921, a German physiologist previously found that animating the vagus nerve caused the pulse to back off by setting off the arrival of a substance he called Vagusstoff (vagus substance). It was later found that this substance was really acetylcholine—a significant synapse in our sensory system. From that point forward, scientists have found more information about the vagus nerve and the role it plays in various infections and significant frameworks in the body. For instance, electrical incitement of this nerve has been discovered to decrease the pace of epileptic seizures and help with burdensome manifestations. Vagal tone—or how solid your vagus nerve is—can be associated with irritation, resistant framework guideline, digestion, and passionate guideline, which we would all be able to concur are entirely significant.

So what does the vagus nerve mean for psychological wellness? Low vagal tone is related with poor passionate and attentional guideline, aggravation, discouragement, and is even utilized as an estimation for an individual's ability to push. Then, a solid vagal tone is related with the inverse: positive feelings and mental parity. A few investigations have even demonstrated that expanding vagal tone could be useful in treating fixation and certain longings. Knowing this, it may be time—to pay tribute to Mental Health Month—for us all to concentrate up on this significant piece of the body.

Would I Be Able to Fortify My Nagus nerve Without Anyone Else?

Thinking about whether you can reinforce your vagal tone for better wellbeing? You're in karma! Numerous therapists, neuroscientists, and integrative wellbeing specialists state we can take advantage of the intensity of the vagus nerve to improve our emotional wellness. Christopher Bergland in Psychology Today composed that "Vagusstoff (acetylcholine) resembles a sedative that you can self-regulate essentially by taking moderate, profound diaphragmatic breaths."

As it were, the vagus nerve has an inseparable tie to breathing—no big surprise; associating with the breath is an establishing guideline in both yoga and contemplation. Be that as it may, other than breathing, there are a large group of various approaches to give your vagus nerve a truly necessary exercise.

Here are five things that will enable you to battle nervousness and weight on a neurobiological level:

1. Singing and music.

Research demonstrates that singing has an organically alleviating impact, which has an inseparable tie to the vagus nerve. This can be anything from a moderate mantra to reciting to belting out your top pick '90s melody.

2. Giggling.

In studies testing the impacts of vagus nerve incitement on kids with epilepsy, one of the symptoms is wild giggling. And keeping in mind that it is anything but an ideal reaction in a clinical setting, this shows chuckling is related with an expansion in vagal incitement. So chuckle and snicker frequently; there are such huge numbers of demonstrated advantages!

3. Irregular fasting.

A few examinations propose that fasting and dietary limitation can actuate the vagus nerve, and considering the various medical advantages of fasting, it's certainly something to consider.

4. Biofeedback.

Biofeedback, particularly pulse changeability biofeedback, is a stunning kind of innovation that works by showing a visual portrayal of what's going on inside the body. Along these lines, an individual can all the more likely comprehend the physiological impacts of profound breathing or unwinding strategies; the vagus nerve assumes a significant job in breathing guideline and pulse fluctuation, so this can be a fun method to practice it.

5. Cold presentation.

Studies demonstrate that cool presentation causes a move toward parasympathetic sensory system action, which as we probably are aware is adjusted by the vagus nerve. So in the event that you've never investigated the advantages of hot to cold showering, your vagus nerve could be a valid justification to begin.

6. Probiotics.

We definitely realize that the vagus nerve assumes a significant job in the gut-cerebrum pivot. However, on account of science, we presently realize that gut microorganisms can really initiate the vagus nerve. As you can envision, this assumes a significant job in our cerebrum and conduct—on the off chance that you require another motivation to put resources into a viable probiotic.

CHAPTER EIGHT

EXERCISES AND OTHER TECHNIQUES TO REDUCE STRESS, ANXIETY, REGULATE HORMONES, AND STRENGTHEN YOUR IMMUNE SYSTEM

You realize that activity does your body great; however, you're too occupied and worried to fit it into your daily schedule. Hang on a second — there's uplifting news with regards to exercise and stress.

In every way that really matters, any type of movement, from heart invigorating activity to yoga, can go about as a weight reliever. On the probability that you're not a contender or paying little respect to whether you're corroded, you can regardless make a little exercise go far toward weight the board. Find the association among exercise and stress alleviation — and why exercise ought to be a piece of your pressure the executives plan.

How Does Interminable Pressure Influence Your Wellbeing?

The substantial changes that occur during snapshots of stress can be exceptionally useful when they occur for a brief span. Yet, when this occurs for an extensive stretch of time, delivering too many pressure hormones can influence your wellbeing. Medical issues can include:

Stomach-Related Framework

Stomach torments, because of a lull in the rate that the stomach discharges subsequent to eating; additionally loose bowels because of greater movement in the colon.

Heftiness

Increment in craving, which can prompt weight gain. Being overweight or corpulent puts you in danger for diabetes and cardiovascular ailment.

Invulnerable framework

Debilitated invulnerable framework with the goal that you are bound to have colds or different contaminations.

Sensory system

Tension, melancholy, loss of rest, and absence of enthusiasm for physical action. Memory and basic leadership can likewise be influenced.

Cardiovascular framework

Increment in circulatory strain, pulse, and the degree of fats in your blood (cholesterol and triglycerides). Additionally, increment in blood glucose levels, particularly at night, and craving. These are hazard factors for coronary illness, atherosclerosis (solidifying of the veins), stroke, weight, and diabetes.

How Would You Realize When You're Worried?

At the point when you experience transient pressure, you may feel on edge, anxious, occupied, stressed, and compelled. On the off chance that your feeling of anxiety increases or goes on for a more extended time, you may encounter other physical or passionate impacts:

- Fatigue, melancholy
- Chest torment or weight, quick heartbeat
- Dizziness, flimsiness, trouble relaxing
- Irregular menstrual periods, erectile brokenness (weakness), loss of charisma (sex drive)

These manifestations may likewise prompt loss of craving, indulging, and poor rest, all of which can adversely affect your wellbeing. Typically, side effects are minor and might be calmed through adapting abilities, for example, figuring out how to unwind, expelling yourself for a period from the things that worry you, and working out. On the off chance that the side effects are extreme, in any case, you may require therapeutic assistance to discover the wellspring of your pressure and the most ideal approach to oversee it.

Exercise and Stress Help

Exercise expands your general wellbeing and your feeling of prosperity, which places more enthusiasm in your progression consistently. In any case, practice likewise has some immediate pressure busting benefits:

- • It siphons up your endorphins. Physical action helps knock up the creation of your mind's vibe great synapses, called endorphins. Despite the fact that this capacity is regularly alluded to as a sprinter's high, an animating round of tennis or a nature climb likewise can add to this equivalent inclination.

- • It's contemplation moving. After a quick paced round of racquetball or a few laps in the pool, you'll regularly find that you've overlooked the day's disturbances and focused distinctly on your body's developments.

- • As you start to routinely shed your day-by-day strains through development and physical action, you may find that this attention on a solitary assignment, and the subsequent vitality and positive thinking, can enable you to keep quiet and clear in all that you do.

- • It improves your disposition. Normal exercise can build fearlessness, it can loosen up you, and it can bring down the side effects related with mellow despondency and uneasiness. Exercise can likewise improve your rest, which is regularly disturbed by pressure, melancholy, and tension. The advantages of these activities can facilitate your feelings of anxiety and give you a feeling of direction over your body and your life.

Approaches to Relax and Rejuvenate

Stress appears to have turned into a steady factor in the present quick-paced society. Whenever left unchecked, it can unleash destruction upon our wellbeing. Figuring out how to successfully oversee pressure can mean the contrast between being hearty and loaded with life, or getting to be defenseless to ailment and sickness. Stress can debilitate the safe framework and quicken the maturing procedure. The capacity to unwind and revive advances health, essentialness, and life span.

A sound safe framework manages our body's mending procedure and protects it against contaminations and sicknesses. At the point when stress bargains our insusceptible capacity, it can bring about colds, influenza, exhaustion, cardiovascular issue, and untimely maturing. Stress expands pulse, circulatory strain, glucose levels, adrenaline, cortisol, free radicals, and oxidative harm. This starts the "battle or flight" reaction, places undue strain upon the heart, and can likewise expand the sentiments of nervousness and despondency.

Ensuring the safe framework is a crucial piece of living longer, feeling more youthful, and being sound.

Here are ten solid approaches to decrease pressure,

support your resistant framework, and hinder the hands of time:

1. Strolling and Physical Activity (Moving, Planting, Cycling, Swimming, etc.): Ordinary exercise and physical movement fortifies your resistant framework, cardiovascular framework, heart, muscles, and bones. It additionally invigorates the arrival of endorphins, improves mental working, focus/consideration and subjective execution, and brings down cholesterol, pulse, cortisol and different pressure hormones. Three 10-minute exercise sessions during the day are similarly as compelling as one 30-minute exercise, and significantly simpler to fit into a bustling calendar.

2. Yoga and Stretching: The sluggish developments and controlled stances of yoga improves muscle quality, adaptability, scope of movement, balance, breathing, blood flow, mental center, clearness, and tranquility. Extending additionally lessens mental and physical pressure, strain and tension, advances great rest, brings down pulse, and hinders your pulse.

3. Hand Hygiene: The best measure in counteracting the spread of microorganisms that cause diseases is great hand cleanliness. Washing your hands with cleanser and water when you get back home, and consistently before you eat, extraordinarily lessens your introduction to bacterial and viral contaminations. In the event that you can't wash with cleanser and water when you are away from home, convey some liquor based hand wipes with you to control microbial presentation and transmission.

4. Giggling and Humor: There is truth to the platitude that giggling is the best medication. Snickering lessens pressure hormones like adrenaline (epinephrine) and cortisol. It likewise benefits your insusceptible framework by expanding the number and action of Natural Killer T-cells. These cells go about as the principal line of protection against viral assaults and harmed cells. Discover the amusingness in things and take part in exercises that make you giggle to expand your invulnerable capacity and infection obstruction.

5. High Nutrient Diet: Eat nourishments plentiful in cell reinforcements (like nutrients A, C, E and lycopene), omega-3 unsaturated fats, and folate. Cell reinforcements battle and kill free radicals, which are particles that harm cells and cause coronary illness, disease, and untimely maturing. Omega-3 unsaturated fats (a polyunsaturated fat) have calming, cardiovascular-improving and resistant controlling properties. It is useful in anticipating and controlling elevated cholesterol, hypertension, coronary illness, stroke, malignant growth, diabetes, melancholy, incendiary, and auto-insusceptible issue. Folate averts age-related subjective decrease, harm to veins and synapses by bringing down homocysteine levels. It likewise guarantees DNA respectability (significant as we age and when pregnant) and advances solid red platelets.

Superb nourishment hotspots for these supplements are as per the following:

- Antioxidants - pumpkin, sweet potatoes, carrots, kale, grapefruit (red and pink), blueberries, strawberries, watermelon, melon, oranges, peppers (red and green), tomatoes, broccoli, sunflower seeds, almonds and olive oil.

- Omega-3 Fatty Acids - ground flax seeds, pecans, soybeans and pumpkin seeds.

- Folate - dull green verdant vegetables (turnip greens, mustard greens, spinach, romaine lettuce, collard greens, and so forth.), beans, vegetables, asparagus, Brussels sprouts, beets and okra.

6. Music: Tuning in to your preferred music is an extraordinary technique for diminishing pressure and assuaging tension. Your individual inclination in music figures out which sorts of calming sounds will best lessen your strain, circulatory strain, and advance sentiments of serenity. Focus on how you feel when you hear a specific tune or classification of music, and hold tuning in to the ones that produce a loosening-up impact.

7. Rest: Getting enough stable rest profoundly affects your feelings of anxiety, invulnerable capacity, and infection opposition. A ceaseless absence of rest can leave you feeling drowsy, bad-tempered, absentminded, clumsy, and experience issues focusing or adapting to life's day-by-day aggravations. Long haul rest misfortune can likewise bring about coronary illness, stroke, hypertension, sorrow, and uneasiness. Rest time is the point at which your body and safe framework do the vast majority of its fixes and restoration. Endeavor to get 7-8 hours of rest every night. Keep in mind rest and unwinding go inseparably.

8. Positive Thinking: Good faith can balance the negative effect pressure, strain and uneasiness has on your invulnerable framework and prosperity. Regularly, it is the way you see things that decide whether you get overpowered, both rationally and physically. Having an uplifting mentality, finding the positive qualities in what life tosses your direction and taking a gander at the splendid side of things upgrades your capacity to successfully oversee pressure.

9. Tea: Normally, drinking tea for the duration of the day can help reinforce your safe framework and your body's capacity to fend off germs and diseases. Both green and dark teas contain a useful amino corrosive called L-theanine, which can expand the contamination battling limit of gamma delta T cells. L-theanine likewise advances a feeling of unwinding, tranquillity and prosperity by affecting the discharge and grouping of synapses (like dopamine, serotonin and GABA) in the mind.

10. Hydrotherapy: Unwinding in a hot shower soothes sore muscles and joints, decreases pressure and strain, and advances a decent night's rest. Include some mitigating music, delicate lighting and normally scented shower salts, bubble shower/shower froth to make a cheap and advantageous spa involvement in the security of your own home.

To kick you off, attempt this tasty and nutritious formula by Monique N. Gilbert. It's high in cell reinforcements and Omega-3 unsaturated fats.

Banana Strawberry Power Smoothie

- 1 solidified ready banana
- 1 cup strawberries (new or solidified)
- 1/2 cup squeezed orange
- 1/2 cup soymilk
- 2 tablespoons canned pumpkin
- 1 tablespoon ground flax seeds
- 1 tablespoon nectar or veggie lover nectar substitute.

Mix in a nourishment processor or blender for 1-2 minutes, until smooth and rich. Makes around 2-3/4 cups (2 servings)

How Might I Balance My Hormones?

A hormonal irregularity can fundamentally affect state of mind, craving, and by and large wellbeing. A few variables, including maturing, are past an individual's control. Be that as it may, reasonable components, for example, stress and the eating regimen can likewise impact hormone levels.

The endocrine framework circles hormones, which perform different capacities for the duration of the day.

Indeed, even little changes in hormone levels can bring about unfriendly impacts, including additional weight on the body. Indications can deteriorate after some time, and a hormonal irregularity can prompt interminable issues.

For certain individuals, making straightforward way of life changes can re-establish levels of hormones.

The following tips may help:

1.   Get enough rest

Rest might be among the most significant elements for hormonal parity. Levels of certain hormones may rise and fall for the duration of the day because of issues, for example, the nature of rest.

As per an examination in the International Journal of Endocrinology Trusted Source, the antagonistic impacts of rest unsettling influence on hormones may add to:

- obesity
- diabetes
- problems with craving

Normally, getting a full, undisturbed, night's rest may enable the body to manage hormone levels.

2. Stay away from an excessive amount of light around evening time

Introduction to blue light, for example, from phones or PC screens, can disturb the rest cycle. The body reacts to this light as though it were sunshine and alters hormones accordingly.

An investigation in Chronobiology International Trusted Source shows that exposes to any brilliant fake lighting around evening time may befuddle the body, making it smother the hormone melatonin, which can contrarily influence numerous capacities.

Staying away from counterfeit lights may help manage hormones and re-establish a characteristic circadian mood.

3. Oversee pressure

An investigation in the diary Experimental and Clinical Sciences Trusted Source shows a connection between stress, the endocrine framework, and hormone levels. The analysts contend that the connection is solid, with even a low degree of stress causing an endocrine reaction.

Stress prompts an expansion in adrenaline and cortisol. On the off chance that degrees of these hormones are excessively high, it can disturb the general parity and add to variables, for example, stoutness, changes in state of mind, and even cardiovascular issues.

Consequently, it is essential to discover approaches to diminish pressure. An examination in the diary Psychoneuroendocrinology Trusted Source proposes that the straightforward demonstration of tuning in to music decreases pressure, particularly if the individual is aiming to unwind.

4. Exercise

The hormonal impacts of ordinary exercise may anticipate indulging. An examination in the diary Sports Medicine Trusted Source shows that even short exercise sessions help direct hormones that control craving.

Additionally, as an article in BMJ Open Sport and Exercise Medicine Trusted Source calls attention to, ordinary physical action diminishes the danger of insulin opposition, metabolic disorder, and type 2 diabetes.

5. Avoid sugars

Discoveries detailed in Critical Reviews in Clinical Laboratory Sciences Trusted Source bolster the possibility that sugar assumes a job in issues, for example, metabolic malady and insulin opposition.

While solid proof is as yet missing, wiping out sugar from the eating routine may help keep levels of hormones, including insulin, under tight restraints.

A few people keep away from explicit sugars. In any case, ongoing exploration in The Journal of Nutrition Trusted Source found that table sugar, high-fructose corn syrup, and nectar caused comparable reactions. An individual may, hence, benefit from avoiding all sugar, instead of explicit sorts.

6. Eat energizing fats

Energizing fats may help keep up a parity of

hormones associated with hunger, digestion, and feeling full.

An examination in the diary Nutrients Trusted Source recommends that medium-chain unsaturated fats, for example, those found in coconut or red palm oils, may work to control the cells liable for the body's reaction to insulin.

In the meantime, an investigation in the American Journal of Clinical Nutrition Trusted Source found that olive oil may adjust levels of a hormone that controls the craving and invigorates the absorption of fat and protein.

Separate research, in the diary Peptides Trusted Source, indicated comparative outcomes.

7. Eat loads of fiber

Fiber may assume a significant job in gut wellbeing, and it might likewise help direct hormones, for example, insulin.

An examination in the diary Obesity shows that a few sorts of fiber work to adjust levels of different hormones too, which may enable an individual to keep up a solid weight.

8. Eat a lot of greasy fish

The elevated levels of fats in some fish can add to heart and stomach related wellbeing and may likewise profit the cerebrum and focal sensory system.

As an investigation in Frontiers in Psychology Trusted Source shows, eating an eating regimen wealthy in sleek fish may help counteract disposition issue, for example, sorrow and nervousness. Now and again, adding sleek fish to the eating regimen may add to treating the scatters.

The omega-3s in greasy fish may assume an especially noteworthy job in adjusting disposition, however completely understanding the connection will require further research.

9. Abstain from indulging

Routinely indulging may prompt metabolic issues in the long haul; however, an investigation in Obesity found that even momentary gorging changes coursing levels of fats and builds oxidative pressure.

The scientists additionally point to an expansion in ceramides, which are fat cells in the skin, taking note that a critical increment may advance insulin opposition. They call for further investigation into this territory.

10. Drink green tea

Green tea is for the most part stimulating refreshment, containing cancer prevention agents and intensifies that lift metabolic wellbeing.

A survey in the American Journal of Clinical Nutrition Trusted Source shows a connection between green tea and decreased fasting insulin levels.

The cell reinforcements in the tea may likewise help oversee oxidative pressure.

11. Stop smoking tobacco

Tobacco smoke may upset degrees of a few hormones.

For instance, as indicated by an examination in the International Journal of General Medicine Trusted Source, the smoke may modify thyroid hormone levels, invigorate pituitary hormones, and even raise levels of steroid hormones, for example, cortisol, which is connected to pressure.

For Females

The following tips may help balance hormones in females:

Be careful about dairy items

Dairy is a significant wellspring of supplements for some individuals. Nonetheless, females worried about degrees of conceptive hormones may wish to utilize alert, particularly before expending cream or yogurt.

An investigation in The Journal of Nutrition Trusted Source shows that eating dairy can lessen levels of some defensive hormones. What's more, the creators point to a relationship between eating cream and yogurt and missing ovulation. The connection is vague, and the specialists call for further investigations.

Think about enhancements and elective drugs

There is some proof that elective treatments or enhancements may address some hormonal issues. For example, an examination in Complementary Therapies in Medicine Trusted Source found that a Chinese home grown treatment routine brought about multiplied pregnancy rates, contrasted with Western, medicate based treatment, among female members with barrenness.

Another investigation, in the Avicenna Journal of Phytomedicine Trusted Source, reports that Nigella Sativa, known as dark seeds or fennel blossom seeds, helped raise estrogen levels in a creature model.

In the event that reviews in people affirm these discoveries, the enhancement might be helpful for individuals experiencing menopause.

For Guys

The following tip may profit guys:

Consider wiping out liquor

While most specialists believe drinking modest quantities helps to invigorate eating regimen, an examination in the diary BMJ Open found that even unobtrusive liquor utilization may upset hormone levels in youngsters. The scientists noticed an association between ordinary liquor utilization and decreased sperm quality, just as changes in testosterone levels.

For guys with worries about hormone levels, it might be ideal to confine or kill liquor utilization.

Tips for kids

The next may profit kids, specifically:

Cut back on handled starches

Sugars are not by any means the only dietary guilty party with regards to insulin obstruction. Prepared starches, for example, white bread items and heated products, may likewise add to insulin opposition.

An examination in the diary Mediators of Inflammation Trusted Source found a connection between eating regimens high in refined sugars and insulin obstruction in youngsters. Disposing of prepared carbs may help diminish this hazard.

Takeaway

Hormones influence a wide scope of substantial capacities, and even little awkward nature can have huge outcomes. For certain individuals, making dietary and way of life changes can re-establish a solid equalization.

Musculoskeletal Framework

At the point when the body is focused on, muscles worry. Muscle strain is just about a reflex response to push — the body's method for guarding against damage and agony.

With unexpected beginning pressure, the muscles worry at the same time, and after that discharge their strain when the pressure passes. Interminable pressure makes the muscles in the body be in a pretty much consistent condition of guardedness. At the point when muscles are rigid and tense for extensive stretches of time, this may trigger different responses of the body and even advance pressure related issue. For instance, both pressure type cerebral pain and headache migraine are related with constant muscle strain in the territory of the shoulders, neck, and head. Musculoskeletal torment in the low back and furthest points has additionally been connected to pressure, particularly employment stress.

A large number of people experience the ill effects of ceaseless difficult conditions optional to musculoskeletal issue. Regularly, however not generally, there might be damage that sets off the constant difficult state. What decides if a harmed individual proceeds to experience the ill effects of ceaseless torment is the manner by which they react to the damage. People who are frightful of torment and re-damage, and who look for just a physical reason and solution for the damage, for the most part have a more regrettable recuperation than people who keep up a specific degree of moderate, doctor regulated action.

Unwinding systems and different pressure calming exercises and treatments have been shown to viably diminish muscle strain, decline the frequency of certain pressure related issue, for example, cerebral pain, and increase the feeling of prosperity. For the individuals who create interminable agony conditions, stress-soothing exercises have been shown to improve state of mind and day-by-day work.

Respiratory Framework

Be aware that the respiratory framework, after supplying oxygen to cells, expels carbon dioxide out of the body. When inhaling occurs through the nose, it passes through the larynx in the throat, and it passes through the trachea down into the lungs (through the bronchi). However, the bronchioles, for flow, carry oxygen to red platelets.

Stress and forceful feelings can give respiratory side effects, for example, brevity of breath and fast breathing, as the aviation route between the nose and the lungs tightens. For individuals without respiratory infection, this is commonly not an issue, as the body can deal with the extra work to inhale easily, yet mental stressors can worsen breathing issues for individuals with previous respiratory ailments, for example, asthma and interminable obstructive aspiratory ailment (COPD; incorporates emphysema and ceaseless bronchitis).

A few examinations demonstrate that an intense

pressure — for example, the passing of a friend or family member — can really trigger asthma assaults. Likewise, the quick breathing — or hyperventilation — brought about by pressure can expedite a fit of anxiety in somebody inclined to fits of anxiety.

Working with an analyst to create unwinding, breathing, and other subjective conduct methodologies can help.

Cardiovascular

The heart and veins contain the two components of the cardiovascular framework that work together in giving sustenance and oxygen to the organs of the body. The movement of these two components is likewise planned in the body's reaction to stretch. Intense pressure — stress that is transitory or momentary, for example, complying with time constraints, being trapped in rush hour gridlock or abruptly pummeling on the brakes to maintain a strategic distance from a mishap — causes an expansion in pulse and more grounded constrictions of the heart muscle, with the pressure hormones — adrenaline, noradrenaline and cortisol — going about as couriers for these impacts. Likewise, the veins that immediate blood to the huge muscles and the heart expand, consequently expanding the measure of blood siphoned to these pieces of the body and hoisting circulatory strain. This is otherwise called the "battle or flight" reaction. When the intense pressure scene has passed, the body comes back to its ordinary state.

CONCLUSION

Incessant pressure, or a steady pressure experienced over a drawn out timeframe, can add to long haul issues for heart and veins. The steady and continuous increment in pulse, and the raised degrees of stress hormones and of circulatory strain, can negatively affect the body. This long haul continuous pressure can build the hazard for hypertension, coronary failure, or stroke.

Rehashed intense pressure and diligent interminable pressure may likewise add to irritation in the circulatory framework, especially in the coronary courses, and this is one pathway that is thought to bind worry to cardiovascular failure. It likewise creates the impression that how an individual reacts to pressure can influence cholesterol levels.

The hazard for coronary illness related with pressure seems to vary for ladies, contingent upon whether the lady is pre or postmenopausal. Levels of estrogen in premenopausal ladies seem to help veins react better during pressure, along these lines helping their bodies to all the more likely handle pressure and protecting them against coronary illness. Postmenopausal ladies lose this degree of security because of loss of estrogen, along these lines putting them at more serious hazard for the impacts of weight on coronary illness.

Endocrine

At the point when somebody sees a circumstance to challenge, undermining or wild, the cerebrum starts a course of occasions including the hypothalamic-pituitary-adrenal (HPA) hub, which is the essential driver of the endocrine pressure reaction. This, in the end, result in an expansion in the generation of steroid hormones called glucocorticoids, which incorporate cortisol, frequently alluded to as the "stress hormone".

The HPA Hub

During times of pressure, the nerve center, a gathering of cores that interfaces the mind and the endocrine framework, flag the pituitary organ to deliver a hormone, which thus flag the adrenal organs, situated over the kidneys, to build the generation of cortisol. Cortisol expands the degree of vitality fuel accessible by assembling glucose and unsaturated fats from the liver. Cortisol is regularly created in fluctuating levels for the duration of the day, commonly expanding in fixation after arousing and gradually declining for the duration of the day, giving a day-by-day cycle of vitality. During an unpleasant occasion, an expansion in cortisol can furnish the vitality required to manage drawn-out or extraordinary test.

Stress and wellbeing

Glucocorticoids, including cortisol, are significant for managing the invulnerable framework and diminishing irritation. While this is important during upsetting or undermining circumstances where damage may bring about expanded insusceptible framework enactment, incessant pressure can bring about impeded correspondence between the safe framework and the HPA pivot. This disabled correspondence has been connected to the future improvement of various physical and psychological well-being conditions, including constant exhaustion, metabolic issue (e.g., diabetes, corpulence), discouragement, and safe issue.

Gastrointestinal

The gut has a huge number of neurons which can work reasonably freely and are in steady correspondence with the mind disclosing the capacity to feel "butterflies" in the stomach. Stress can influence this mind gut correspondence, and may trigger agony, swelling, and other gut inconvenience to be felt all the more effectively. The gut is likewise occupied by a great many microorganisms which can impact its wellbeing and the mind's wellbeing which can affect the capacity to think and influence feelings. Stress is related to changes in gut microorganisms which thus can impact state of mind. Subsequently, the gut's nerves and microscopic organisms emphatically impact the mind and the other way around.

Early life stress can change the improvement of the sensory system just as how the body responds to pressure. These progressions can expand the hazard for later gut sicknesses or dysfunctioning.

Throat

At the point when focused on, people may eat substantially more or significantly less than expected. More or various nourishments, or an expansion in the utilization of liquor or tobacco, can bring about indigestion or heartburn. Stress or depletion can likewise build the seriousness of consistently happening acid reflux torment. An uncommon instance of fits in the throat can be set off by exceptional pressure and can be effectively confused with a coronary failure. Stress likewise may make gulping nourishments troublesome or increase the measure of air that is gulped, which expands burping, gassiness, and swelling.

Stomach

Stress may make torment, swelling, sickness, and other stomach distress felt all the more effectively. Spewing may happen if the pressure is extreme enough. Besides, stress may cause a superfluous increment or lessening in hunger.